LETTERS FROM A FRIEND
A Sibling's Guide for Coping and Grief

Erika Barber, C.C.L.S., B.S.

Death, Value and Meaning Series
Series Editor: John D. Morgan

Baywood Publishing Company, Inc.
AMITYVILLE, NEW YORK

Copyright © 2003 by Baywood Publishing Company, Inc., Amityville, New York

All rights reserved. No part of this book may be reproduced or utilized in any form or by any means, electronic or mechanical, including photo-copying, recording, or by any information storage or retrieval system, without permission in writing from the publisher. Printed in the United States of America on acid-free recycled paper.

Baywood Publishing Company, Inc.
26 Austin Avenue
Amityville, NY 11701
(800) 638-7819
E-mail: baywood@baywood.com
Web site: baywood.com

ISBN: 0-89503-248-1 (paper)

Dedication

This guide is dedicated to the memory of my sister
ANDREA MARTINA NEUGEBAUER

During her life, Andrea had two dreams: to become an elementary school teacher and to make a positive difference in the lives of children and young adults. Andrea died before she could become a teacher. Yet, it is my hope that this guide may help fulfill Andrea's other precious dream.

I love you, Andrea

Erika Barber / Letters From a Friend
P.O. Box 59069
Schaumburg, Illinois 60159

Throughout this guide, names of people and character descriptions, as well as personal situations and experiences, have been changed to protect privacy rights.

Table of Contents

My Sibling's Illness/Injury 1

Dying and Hospice 6

My Past Death Experiences 14

My Sibling's Death 19

Death Services/Ceremonies 28

Sympathy Cards/SIB-A-THY Card Program 35

Visiting My Sibling's Body 39

Returning to School 42

My Religion and My God 47

Grief Feelings 52

Denial 54

Anger 57

Sadness 66

It's Not Fair 71

Guilt/If I Had Only 74

Afraid 80

Joy/Happiness 88

The Game of Survival 91

My Family 100

Police and the Law 113

Newspapers, TV, and the Media 116

My Sibling's Friends 117

Dreams and Nightmares 123

Anniversaries and "Firsts" 128

Identity 134

Emotional Support 140

Surviving My Future 149

Shapes of Survival: A Game of Reflection 153

Forgiveness 158

Pen Pal Program 162

Parents, Caregivers, and Professionals 165

Blank Schedule and Calendar 167

Index 169

Within my eight years of experience as a Child Life Specialist at Loyola University Medical Center near Chicago and the University of Wisconsin Children's Hospital in Madison, I have had opportunities to develop relationships with many ill and injured children and adolescents. I have been able to function as an emotional support person as patients, siblings, parents, and caregivers adapt to and cope with hospitalizations, illnesses, or injuries. Many times I have been fortunate to be invited into families as children or adolescents are dying and even after patient death.

Developing *Letters from a Friend: A Sibling's Guide for Coping and Grief* was, truthfully, a very therapeutic project as I shared my thoughts and feelings related to my own sibling's illness, her death, and my survival. Through this project, I have come to understand more fully my own feelings and thoughts, my values, and my appreciation of the unique sibling relationship.

I have always felt a special bond with the patients' brothers and sisters—a bond which unites all of us who have experienced sibling illness, injury, or death. And so, this guide is written for those brothers and sisters so that we can, together and despite these challenges, celebrate our sibling-hood.

Acknowledgments

Thank you to:

Kathy Andrews-Wallensack for sharing your zest for humor and life and your divine spirit of friendship.

Craig Brodsky for your valuable computer lessons and emotional support so that I was able to type this guide.

Stuart Cohen and your remarkable staff at Baywood, especially Julie Krempa, Bobbi Olszewski, and Joi Tamber-Brooks whose patience, advice, and ongoing commitment made my dream possible.

Bob Kemp for your legal insight and direction.

Andrea Leppert for taking hold of my hand while we waited together on my living room couch so many years ago and for never letting go since. You are the closest bond to sister-hood I have.

Shari Lichtenstein for your encouragement and advice from your perspective as an author and for your emotional support as a friend.

Susan Medina for your wisdom of the human heart and for your role as my spiritual mentor.

John D. Morgan, Ph.D., my editor, for your professional guidance and management. Thank you for believing in this guide and, in doing so, enabling this one sibling survivor to reach out to so many others.

My parents, *Theresia and William Ruppel* and *John and Marilyn Neugebauer.* You all have taught me so much about emotional strength, about forgiveness, and about enduring love.

Amie, Brooke, Cheryl, Jan, Jay, Jill, Karen, Kerry, Laurel, Sarah, and Susan. Thank you all for talking and listening about Andrea's death, and thereby celebrating and acknowledging her life . . . thank you for allowing me to feel whatever emotion I was feeling without judgment . . . thanks for sharing the experiences and creating the memories of life which helped me to define myself as a "survivor."

My God, who kept loving me when I walked away and throughout my journey back to spirituality.

And, finally . . .

to *you*, surviving brother or sister. Thank you for allowing me to share Andrea's life and death with you. Remember, you are special. You always will be.

Dear Mom, Dad, Caregiver, Professional,

Welcome to *Letters from a Friend: A Sibling's Guide for Coping and Grief*!

Letters from a Friend is more than just an exercise in creative writing and drawing for a child or teen sibling. It is a teacher, as it provides opportunities for experimentation and learning about one's own world. It is a guide, as it allows self-exploration and self-discovery within a variety of activities and may foster the creation of a book as a sibling completes these activities. Most importantly, it is a supportive friend, as it shares feelings and a story, yet allows another's feelings and story to be shared.

The guide was specifically designed for the special group of child and adolescent "survivors," to encourage expression of their grief as a sibling is dying and after sibling death. Grief is a very personal experience for everyone, so children and teens will likely grieve differently from one another, regardless of their ages.

There is also a section at the end of this guide *for parents, caregivers and professionals!* Suggestions for utilizing this guide and recommendations on assisting the child or teen author are provided for you.

Although *Letters from a Friend* offers activities which encourage the expression of various emotions, experiences, and beliefs, each author may determine which activities to include in his or her own special book. Throughout the guide, there is narrative or explanations. There are also activity pages.

Child care professionals may select specific pages or sections of this guide to facilitate and assess a child or teen's grieving process while a sibling is dying or after the death of a sibling. Therefore, *Letters from a Friend* has great clinical therapeutic benefits. Authors are encouraged to share some of the activities with adults they trust in order to gain insight to and emotional support of their thoughts and feelings. However, remember that it is not as important that children or adolescents *share* each feeling with someone, as it is they *express* their feelings (and writing is a great means of expression).

Please be available to answer the child or teen's questions, sympathize with his or her feelings, and listen as the child or teen shares his or her thoughts. If you are unable to be consistently available for the child or teen, an adult with whom he or she trusts and feels comfortable may also function as a support person.

Sharing my experiences and feelings in the text serves, I hope, to both encourage the authors to share their own experiences and feelings as well as to reassure them that it is okay to feel every type of emotion.

This guide may also help the younger child and those children not yet able to understand or interpret the text and its activities. These children may share emotions or write their books with support from child care professionals or consistent adults whom they trust.

Thank you for recognizing the uniqueness of sibling relationships, the importance of sibling coping and grief management, and the celebration of sibling survivors.

Dear Brother or Sister,

Welcome to *Letters from a Friend: A Sibling's Guide for Coping and Grief!*

Letters from a Friend is a special guide *just for you!*

It is special to me, because it is written in memory of my only sister, Andrea. Andrea quickly became very sick and died when I was fifteen years old. In many sections of this guide, I share my story about my sister. I also share my story and my feelings about Andrea's death and about my life since she died.

Letters from a Friend is a guide, because it may help you share your story and your feelings about your life as your brother or sister is dying or since your sibling died. As you write and draw pictures about your story and feelings, this guide may also help you create your own special book!

There are many parts of this guide just for you to read. There are also activity pages. You may need additional pages of paper to complete some of the activities.

You will be the author and decide what your book will look like, the length of your chapters, and which creative pictures and activities to include. Pages may be removed from this guide to create your own book.

There may be activities or sections of this guide about feelings, experiences, or beliefs which are different from your own feelings, experiences or beliefs, so you may decide not to use them in your book. You may choose activities from different sections to create your own chapters.

Since this will be a book written by you and for you, you may decide to share it with a special someone or just with yourself. Within the guide, I encourage you to share *some* of the activities with an adult you trust. Look for this reminder before you begin an activity. Even the letters you may write as activities in the guide may be shared with someone or kept as a part of your special book. Within some letter writing activities, you may not feel as if you are writing a "letter from a friend." That's O.K. All of the letter writing activities are important and may, like the other activities, help you express your thoughts and feelings. (And, there are many letters you may write *as* a friend *to* a friend!)

So, this is where your story begins! You are special!

My book is dedicated to _____

Andrea's Story

Andrea was my only sister. In fact, she was my only sibling.

Shortly after her twentieth birthday, Andrea became unhealthy. Yet, her illness could not be seen on X-rays or with microscopes. Andrea's illness was emotional. It was inside her thoughts and feelings. The illness was called "severe depression." Most people do not need to get medicines or visit doctors because they feel sad or depressed. Most people do not feel sad for a very long time.

Andrea felt depressed for many months. My sister even wanted to die because of her illness.

For awhile, Andrea stayed in a hospital. She had many special doctors and took different medicines to help her become healthy again. Yet, the severe depression did not go away.

My Sibling's Illness/Injury

HOSPITAL PHOTOGRAPHS

Your brother or sister may be or may have been hospitalized because of his or her illness or injury.

On this page, place photos or draw pictures of hospital rooms, units, and areas you have seen or of people you have met while visiting your hospitalized brother or sister.

2 / LETTERS FROM A FRIEND

VISITING MY HOSPITALIZED BROTHER/SISTER

Sometimes people look different when they are patients in a hospital, especially if they have injuries or if they have been sick for a long time. If you have visited your sibling in the hospital, draw a picture or place a photo of your hospitalized brother or sister. If you have not visited your brother or sister in the hospital, you may ask an adult who has visited to complete this activity.

If you are not able to visit your brother or sister in the hospital, there are still ways to communicate with him or her!

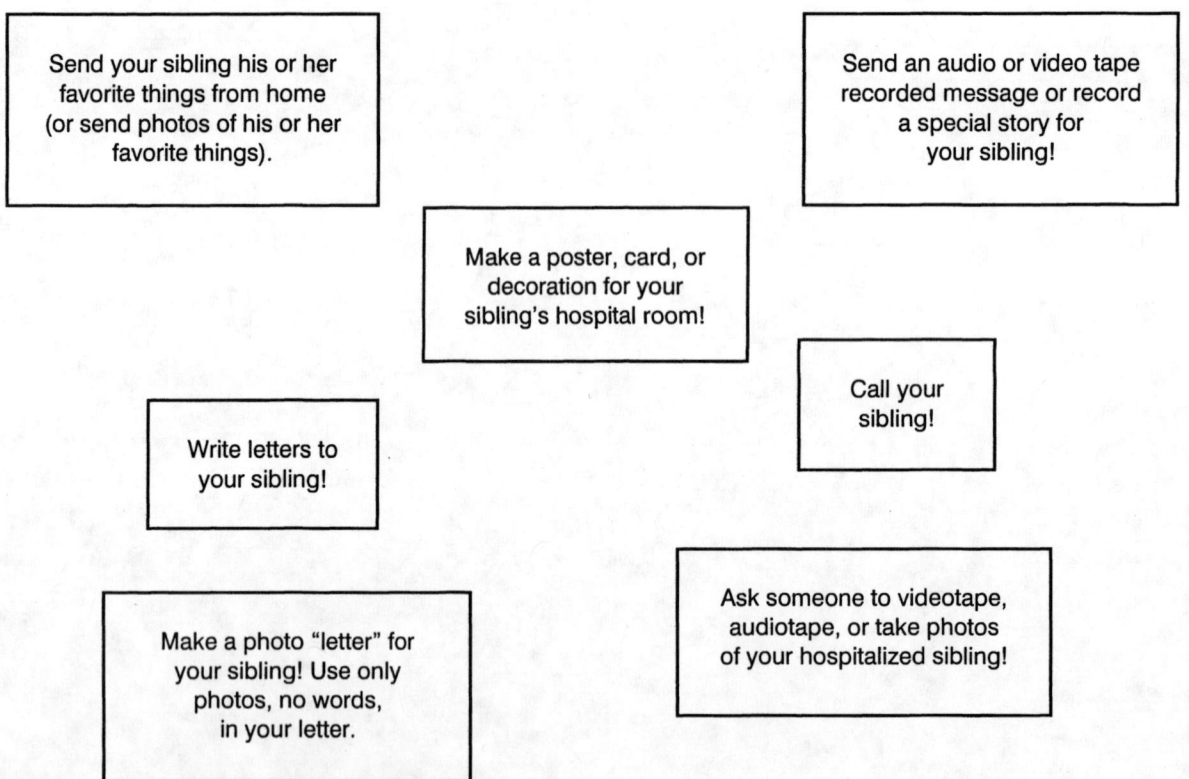

MY SIBLING'S ILLNESS/INJURY

The name of my sibling's illness/injury is _____.

My sibling got the illness/injury when he/she was _____ years old.

I was _____ years old when my sibling got the illness/injury.

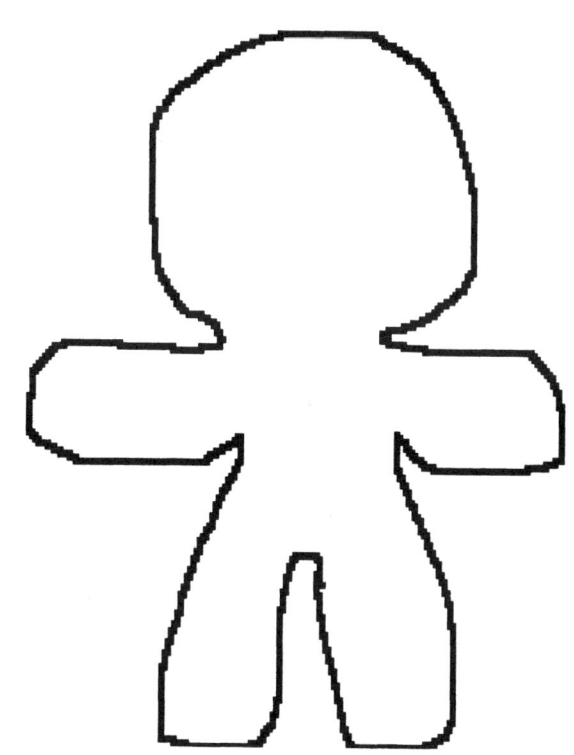

Design this paper person to have the same illness or injury as your sibling. If the illness or injury is unable to be seen, imagine what it would look like. Then, complete your design.

Ask a medical person for gauze coverings, plastic tubing, or other hospital things you may need to complete this activity.

> Remember:
> Your sibling's illness/injury is not a punishment for anything bad which you, your sibling, or anyone else did!

4 / LETTERS FROM A FRIEND

Write a letter to your sibling's illness or injury.

> Remember:
> You may share your letter with someone or just with yourself!

Sometimes, the people in your family may have different feelings about your sibling's illness or injury. You may feel sad. Your mother may feel guilt. Your brother may feel anger.

Imagine: You and your family are on PLANET ILLNESS/INJURY.

Draw a ♥ on a "feeling circle" to show where you are on PLANET ILLNESS/INJURY.
Write the name of each person in your family on a "feeling circle" to show where he or she is on PLANET ILLNESS/INJURY.

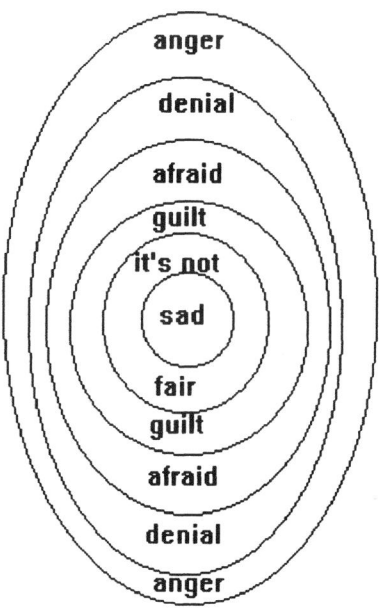

Dying and Hospice

Sometimes, when an illness or injury is not healing and a person is dying, the person may be able to go home instead of staying in a hospital. Nurses and medical people may visit the dying person at his or her home to give medicine or other medical care. This care is called "hospice." Hospice care is not given to help an illness or injury heal. It is given to help the dying person feel more comfortable, especially if the person is very sick or is feeling pain. There are also special hospice buildings where dying people may get hospice care.

Some dying people die at their homes or in hospice care buildings instead of in hospitals. The dying person may like being at home or in a special hospice building better than being in a hospital.

When hospice care is given in homes, some families think their homes look more like hospitals! Sometimes, there are I.V. machines, hospital beds, and visiting medical people. Family routines and plans may change when a person is dying at home.

If your sibling has or had hospice care at home, draw a picture about how your home or your family changed.

If your sibling has or had hospice care in a special hospice building, draw a picture of the building. (You may draw a picture of the inside or outside of the hospice building.)

Since your brother or sister had hospice care, what new rules does or did your family have?

1.

2.

3.

4.

5.

Write your own "Hospice Rules."

1.	4.
2.	5.
3.	6.

Share your rules with someone you trust.

There are many ways you can help your dying brother or sister. You may do the activities with or for your sibling.

Share your ideas with an adult in your family or with a medical person who knows what your brother or sister is able to do. Your sibling may also want to choose which activities to do.

> Remember:
> Your sibling may know you are near, even if he or she is not able to see or talk to you!

If your brother or sister can
See:

You can:

- Blow bubbles
- Make mobiles, posters or other decorations for your sibling's room
- Decorate your sibling's room with family photos, pictures of pets or get well cards
- Rent your sibling's favorite movie
- Polish your sibling's nails or design a new hair style for him or her

If your brother or sister can
Hear:

You can:

- Talk to your sibling about school, his or her friends and your feelings
- Read articles or books to your sibling
- Play your sibling's favorite music for him or her
- Read your sibling's mail to him or her
- Sing to your sibling

If your brother or sister can
Feel or Touch:

You can:

- Massage your sibling with lotion
- Touch your sibling with soft objects (like washcloths and stuffed animals)
- Play with water, sand, or snow in a basin or bucket

CALENDAR CREATIVITY

At the end of this guide, there is a blank calendar. Make copies of the calendar. Then, complete some of these projects:

> Remember:
> An adult family member or a medical person may help you with these projects.

- Make an activity calendar for your dying brother or sister. Plan activities which your sibling may do independently *and* activities which you may do with or for your brother or sister.

- Make a calendar which includes special daily messages for your dying brother or sister.

  Post the calendars in a special place, inside your sibling's room, where your brother or sister can see them.

- Make an activity calendar for you! Plan activities which are important to you. Make plans to be with special people. Planning for time to be alone may be important, too.

> Remember:
> It is O.K. to have fun, even though your brother or sister is dying. It is also important to keep doing the things you used to do, like being with friends and going to school. Planning may help you feel more calm and in control of your life.

- Make a calendar which includes names of the medical tests and other treatments scheduled for your brother or sister. Write the times the medical procedures will happen.

> You may feel better knowing what your brother or sister is doing, especially if you are not able to be with him or her.

10 / LETTERS FROM A FRIEND

Where do you think your brother or sister will die?
Draw a picture of the place.

How do you think your brother or sister will look when he or she dies?

> Share your drawing and your thoughts with an adult you trust.

Who do you think will be with your brother or sister when he or she dies?

WRITE A LETTER TO YOUR DYING BROTHER OR SISTER

Share your thoughts and feelings. Describe the things you like about your sibling and the things you will miss about your brother or sister after he or she has died.

> Remember:
> Share your letter with an adult you trust before sharing it with your sibling, or you may share your letter just with yourself.

Draw a picture or place a photo of your dying brother or sister.

> Remember:
> Your sibling is still your sibling, even if he or she looks different!

Sometimes, after a death, there are special death services or ceremonies. During death services or ceremonies, people may pray for or say "good-bye" to the dead person or thing. Different religions and different families plan different kinds of death services and ceremonies. Death services and ceremonies may happen at funeral homes, churches, temples, family homes, or at other places. Ask an adult in your family about the death services or ceremonies which may be planned for your dying brother or sister.

Sometimes, dying people and their families plan for death. Death planning may seem strange, but it may help people feel more in control of their lives. Some people may feel afraid to plan for death, especially if they do not believe that death will happen.

Before you begin this activity, discuss this activity with an adult in your family and with your dying brother or sister.

If your dying sibling does want to plan for his or her death, you may want to ask him or her:

1. What times and places would you like your death services or ceremonies to occur? What special events or activities would you like planned for your death services or ceremonies?

2. What clothes would you like to wear at your death services or ceremonies?

3. Do you want some of your favorite toys, books, or other things with you at your death services or ceremonies?
   Describe some of the things:

4. Who would you like to invite to your death services or ceremonies?

5. What would you want people to do or say at your death services or ceremonies? (Your brother or sister may want to write a speech, poem, or story to be read at the services or ceremonies.)

> When you have completed this activity, share it with an adult in your family.

If you cannot be with your sibling when he or she dies, it may help to have someone special tell you about your sibling's death.

Who should tell you about your sibling's death?
Write the names of three people.

> Share this activity with the three people on your list.

1)

2)

3)

How should the people on your list tell you that your brother or sister has died?

Where would you want to be when you are told that your sibling died?

My Past Death Experiences

Remember your pets that died.

Share something about the lives or deaths of three different pets.

```
┌─────────────────────┐          ┌─────────────────────┐
│  paste pet photo here│         │  paste pet photo here│
│                     │          │                     │
│                     │          │                     │
│                     │          │                     │
└─────────────────────┘          └─────────────────────┘

           ┌─────────────────────┐
           │  past pet photo here│
           │                     │
           │                     │
           │                     │
           └─────────────────────┘
```

Draw a picture of a pet's death services or ceremonies.

Death happens to every living thing. Sometimes, people may know when someone or something will die. Other times, people or things die suddenly.

Until I was seven years old, I never knew any person who had died. My parents told me when older people who had lived in our neighborhood died. They also told me when one of my cousins died, but I had never met her. When I was seven years old, I understood that people die. I understood that *other* people die, but people who I did know or kids who were my age could not die. I believed death only happened after someone had lived for a long time.

SHARE ONE OF YOUR FIRST EXPERIENCES WHEN A PERSON DIED

What did you understand about death from the experience?

RAYE

Raye taught me a lot more about death when I was in second grade.

She was a blonde-haired, brown-eyed, and freckled-faced girl who sat across from me in Mrs. J's class. During a spelling test one day, I saw Raye copying off my paper. "Please don't tell Mrs. J!" Raye begged. I didn't tell.

A few days after the spelling test, Raye wasn't in class. Mrs. J told us children about the accident. Raye was crossing the street, on her way home from school, and a car drove over her. Raye died in the street on a rainy spring day.

Someone who was my age had died! I knew why. I believed Raye died because she had done a bad thing. She cheated on the spelling test and dying was her punishment. I was wrong.

Death is not a punishment.

Write about the death of someone your age. Share your feelings about the death.

Remember your experiences with death services or ceremonies. Share your feelings about them.
　　Sometimes I felt confused speaking with people about death.

Some people may feel afraid or nervous talking about death. After someone or something dies, some people may not want to talk about the death at all. Other people may use different and sometimes strange words and phrases to explain death.

Instead of telling me that a person "died," I remember:

People saying	I understood
He "passed away."	He fainted.
We "lost her."	We should look for her!
He "went on a vacation."	He will be back when his vacation is over.
She "is sleeping."	She will wake up soon.
He "left us."	We must have done something bad, so he left us! Maybe he will come back if we tell him "We're sorry."
She's "gone."	She will come back.

How was death explained to you? What did you understand about death from the explanations?

My Sibling's Death

There are still times when Andrea's death seems like a fantasy, as if it never really happened. There are moments when I think about my sister, and it seems as if I cannot remember some things about her. I still remember what happened on the day she died, and it seems more like a terrible dream instead of the day which changed my life forever.

I do hope that by sharing my thoughts and feelings with you, I will remember many more things about my relationship with Andrea before she died. I also hope, that as you complete the activities in this guide and share your feelings, thoughts and memories, you too will discover your special sibling relationship, because that is something which never truly dies.

December 17, 1983

I was fifteen years old. Andrea was twenty years old. Christmas was the next week.

I woke up to the sound of holiday carols on my radio alarm clock. School was closed for Christmas vacation and, even though it was Saturday, I had to wake up early. My mom worked at a drapery business. She sewed curtains, and I collected pins and sewing needles from the floor for 50 cents plus free cookies.

On that day, my mother and I quietly showered, quietly got dressed, and quietly ate breakfast, because Andrea was still sleeping. She had been working late the night before and, on that Saturday, had an early appointment with her hospital counselor. We didn't wake her to say, "Good-bye." Instead, we left the house, quietly.

11:32 a.m.

The phone rang. Mom answered it. I knew from the tone of my mother's voice, something bad had happened.

"It's Andrea," was all she said.

I sat in the back seat of the car as my mother's boss drove. My fingers felt cold, and I could feel my heart pounding inside my sweater. The ride home seemed longer than ever, and I thought about jumping from the car and running the rest of the way.

My mother's voice was loud and her face looked pale as she explained what had happened.

Andrea never went to her counseling appointment. My dad wanted to remind her to go to the appointment. He tried to call her many times that morning. Dad rode the train to work that Saturday so

Andrea could use his car, and she did use it, but not to drive anywhere. My neighbor heard Dad's car engine as it sputtered and clanged in the cold winter air of our closed garage. She found Andrea.

Andrea was sitting in the driver's seat with her eyes closed.

From three blocks away I saw the flashing lights, the ambulances, and the crowd of neighbors in front of our house. From the edge of our driveway I saw Dad's car. It was parked in the garage and the doors were open. Andrea was in the ambulance and, before I could see her, the sirens sounded and she was driven away.

ANDREA'S DEATH

Mom and Dad drove to the hospital. I waited at home. A neighbor waited with me. She washed dishes and talked about kitchen safety instead of about Andrea. A friend came over and sat with me on the sofa. We sat together, waiting.

"I know she's dead," I said, without feeling any emotion at all.

Then the phone rang. It was Dad. The neighbor said a few "uh-huhs" and "ummms," and I walked slowly to her. I looked into my neighbor's eyes and, for a moment, we stared at each other.

. . . "Andrea died," the neighbor said through her tangled lips. "She breathed in too much poison gas from the car's exhaust. . . ."

I reached for her as my body fell, crashing to the floor. At the same time, it seemed that my whole world, everything I had known, crashed around me as well.

Some people use the phrase "committed suicide" when they describe Andrea's death. I don't, though. To me, the phrase "committed suicide" sounds as if my sister "committed" a crime. Andrea wasn't a criminal. She chose to die because she was emotionally unhealthy.

MY SIBLING'S DEATH

> Remember:
> It may be helpful to share these activities with an adult you trust.

How old were you when your brother or sister died? _____

How old was your brother or sister when he or she died? _____

DRAW DRAW DRAW DRAW DRAW DRAW DRAW DRAW DRAW DRAW DRAW DRAW
Draw with markers, crayons, or charcoal sticks.

What do you think happened to your brother or sister before he or she died?
DRAW a picture about it.

WRITE: _____
_____
_____
_____
_____

Draw a picture of the place your brother or sister died. If you do not know, draw a picture of the place you think your sibling died.

Write about the day your brother or sister died.

You may share: Why your sibling died or why you think he or she died.
When and where your sibling died or when and where you think your sibling died.
How you knew or were told that your brother or sister died.
Where you were when your brother or sister died.

> **Remember:**
> It may be helpful to share this activity with an adult you trust.

HER BODY

I had never seen a dead person until I saw my sister.

She was lying on a cold metal table in a small room near the hospital's emergency entrance. Andrea's hands and face were very white and her body was warm and limp. Her hand hung down when I lifted and shook her arm. I was trying to wake my sister, or see if she was faking sleep. She wasn't faking though, and she wasn't asleep. Andrea's body was dead.

I still remember the clothes Andrea was wearing: faded blue jeans, red leather boots, and a green ski jacket. Her red-brown hair was lying across her pale face. Andrea rarely wore make-up.

There were no broken bones, and there wasn't any blood. Andrea's dead body did not look like dead bodies I had seen in horror movies, but I still felt afraid, very afraid. I was, afterall, looking at a dead person, and the dead person was my sister.

Draw a picture of what your brother or sister looked like after he or she died.

If you did not see your brother or sister, draw a picture of what you think he or she looked like after death, or ask an adult you trust, who did see your sibling's body, to complete this activity.

> Remember:
> It may be helpful to share your drawing with an adult you trust.

Write three words to describe your sibling or your sibling's body after he or she died.

1. _____ 2. _____ 3. _____

After your brother or sister's death, tell an adult in your family if you do want to have some special time with your sibling's body.

> Remember:
> It is O.K. to touch your sibling's body after he or she died.

Sometimes, photographs of your sibling's body can be taken after he or she has died. The photos may help you grieve and help you share your feelings about your sibling and about his or her death. The photographs might also become very special memories of your brother or sister.

This is a photo of my sibling's body after he or she died. Ask an adult you trust to help you with this activity.

LEAVING THEIR MARKS...

This is an activity to do with an adult you trust.

You will need: Washable tempera paint (you may choose any color or your sibling's favorite color)
　　　　　　　Paper plate
　　　　　　　Clean sponges
　　　　　　　Water

Directions:

1. Pour paint onto paper plate.
2. Dip a sponge in paint.
3. Rub the sponge on the bottom of your sibling's hand or foot until his or her hand or foot is covered with paint.
4. Press this page to your sibling's hand or foot.
5. Remove this page and allow the paint to dry.
6. Use water and the other sponge to clean the paint off your sibling's hand or foot.

You may be very busy during the first few days after your sibling's death. Knowing what will happen during this time may help.

INTERVIEW AN ADULT IN YOUR FAMILY

1. What will be happening during the next few days?

2. What will I be doing during the next few days?

3. What will the other people in my family be doing during the next few days?

4.

5.

6.

7.

8.

9.

10.

You will probably have many kinds of feelings about your sibling's death. On this page, begin a diary to write about all your feelings. You do not need to share your diary with anyone else. Add additional pages as needed.

Date _____

Death Services/Ceremonies

THE WAKE

December 19, 1983

It was 1:04 in the afternoon when Mom, Dad and I walked into the funeral home. Andrea's wake started at 2:00 PM, so we had some time alone with Andrea's body.

The room was small and neat and smelled of the sweet flowers which crowded around the casket. Chairs were placed in rows in the middle of the room, facing the casket.

I remembered how chairs were placed in similar rows, but facing a stage, in my school gymnasium for my fifth grade play. I remembered how the people sat in their chairs, how they stared at the closed curtain, how they waited for the play to begin. I remembered how quiet their voices became once the curtain did open. I wondered if the visitors at Andrea's wake would be the same kind of audience: staring, waiting and listening to the actors: me, Mom, Dad, and Andrea too.

I wished we all were actors and that I was performing in a play. It wasn't a play, though. Andrea's death service was happening, and it was all too real.

There was a heart-shaped flower in the corner of Andrea's casket, just above her head. I saw it from the doorway. Gold lace spelled out "Dear Sister." The flower was from me, although I had never seen it before. I did not help plan Andrea's wake. Nobody asked me if I wanted to help plan it, and I never thought about helping to plan it. If I had helped, I think I would have placed photos of Andrea and me in her casket. I would have wanted something placed with her, something special we once shared.

Mom and Dad left the room, so that I could be alone with my sister's body. I stood beside the large wooden casket and looked down at Andrea's face. Something seemed wrong. The dead person did not look like Andrea! The person's skin looked orange! She had make-up on-lots of make-up-and her hair was straight, not curly like Andrea's.

I thought:

Maybe Andrea's wake was really a play afterall!

Maybe Andrea's death never happened! Maybe I only dreamed that my sister died.

I looked closely at the body, to prove that the dead person was not Andrea. Then, I saw it. As I knelt beside her, I saw Andrea's bump. It was a bump under her nose. I used to tease her about it, because I thought the bump made her nostrils look large. Even though make-up almost covered it, that bump was still there.

The wake lasted for seven hours. Neighbors, family, and her friends came to say "Good-bye" to Andrea.

When strangers hugged me, I didn't feel any emotion. When strangers said, "We're so sorry. Let us know if we can do anything," I smiled, knowing that I would probably never see many of them again.

There were other people who came to the wake, too. My teachers, my friends, and my classmates came to emotionally support *me*! They hugged me. They held my hand. Many of my friends said nothing to me, and even though they were silent, I knew how much they really cared about me.

I felt relieved when people told me, "See you tomorrow." They were telling me there would be a tomorrow and that my life would go on, even though a big part of it-the part with Andrea-would not.

Slowly, the visitors left. Soon, only the three of us stood in that small, neat room. Mom and Dad went to the funeral director's office to talk about the next day's funeral service. I stayed with Andrea's body.

> It was the last time I would be alone with my sister's body.
> It was one of the last times I would see that red-streaked hair, hairs which used to be in *my* hair brush.
> It was one of the last times I would see her long, white fingers, fingers which used to play the violin while I was trying to sleep!
> It was one of the last times I would see . . .
> *that bump.*

I slowly reached out for her fingers and put my hand on hers. Her fingers were hard and she felt cold, very cold.

The small spotlight above Andrea's casket formed shadows across her face. Slowly, I moved my hand up and placed a finger on the bump beneath her nose.

See you tomorrow. I love you, Bignose.

It was the last time I would tease her.

DEATH SERVICES AND CEREMONIES

Sometimes, after a death, there are special death services or ceremonies. During death services or ceremonies, people may pray for or say "good-bye" to the dead person or thing. Different religions and different families plan different kinds of death services and ceremonies. Death services and ceremonies may happen at funeral homes, churches, temples, family homes or at other places.

Ask an adult in your family about the death services or ceremonies which may be planned for your brother or sister who has died.

Draw a picture about the type of death service or ceremony you think your brother or sister would have wanted.

You may share your drawing with your family, with someone else you trust, or just with yourself. Invite friends and family to your sibling's death services or ceremonies. Remember to invite people who will emotionally support *you*! Who will you invite?

1.   4.

2.   5.

3.   6.

What do you think will happen during your sibling's death services or ceremonies?
DRAW a picture about it.

Share your drawing with an adult you trust.

There are many ways you can be involved at your sibling's death services or ceremonies. You may:

- Read a prayer or something your sibling or you wrote.
- Play your sibling's favorite song.
- Choose the clothes your brother or sister will wear at his or her death services or ceremonies.
- Bring special photos of your brother or sister or items which belonged to your sibling to the services or ceremonies for visitors to see.
- Choose a special item to place near your sibling's body.

How would you like to be involved at your sibling's death services or ceremonies?
Write:

_____

_____

_____

_____

_____

_____

> Remember:
> During the death services or ceremonies, it is O.K. to ask for time alone with your sibling's body. It is also O.K. to touch your brother or sister.

Share your ideas with an adult in your family.

NO!NO!NO!NO!NO!NO!NO!NO!NO!NO!NO!NO!NO!NO!NO!NO!NO!NO!NO!NO!NO!

It is O.K. if you do not want to be involved at your sibling's death services or ceremonies. It is O.K. if you do not want to go to the death services or ceremonies. It may be helpful to understand your reasons for these decisions.

I do not, or did not, want to go to or be involved at my brother or sister's death services or ceremonies, because . . . _____

_____

_____

_____

> You may want to ask an adult to photograph your sibling's death services or ceremonies, if you do not go. Photographs can be saved until you are ready to see or talk about them.

32 / LETTERS FROM A FRIEND

Sometimes sign-in books are used at death services or ceremonies. In the book, visitors sign their names or write special messages to the dead person's family.

On this page, begin a sign-in book, just for *you*! Visitors who come to your sibling's death services or ceremonies to emotionally support you may sign their names or write you special messages. You may even decorate these sign-in pages.

> Remember:
> Bring your sign-in book to your brother's or sister's death services or ceremonies. Place your sign-in book where visitors will see it.

_____'s Death Services or Ceremonies
    Sibling's Name

My Sign-In Book

*Date*_____

SHARE YOUR MEMORIES OF YOUR BROTHER'S OR SISTER'S DEATH SERVICES OR CEREMONIES

Write about what you did during the death services or ceremonies. What were some of your feelings during the death services or ceremonies?

What do you remember about your brother's or sister's death services or ceremonies?
Draw a picture about one of your memories.

If you did not go . . .

　　ask an adult who went to your sibling's death services or ceremonies to draw the picture.

Write a story-poem about your brother's or sister's death services or ceremonies.

Written by: _____

Sympathy Cards/SIB-A-THY® Card Program

Many times, after a death, people send sympathy cards to the deceased's family members. Sympathy cards help people express their feelings about a death.

There are many different kinds of sympathy cards. Some of the cards have religious or spiritual messages. Some cards have no printed messages, so that the person sending the card may write his or her own words.

After my sister died, the most beautiful card was sent from one of Andrea's college friends. The card was beautiful, because of its message. Mostly, it was beautiful, because it was just for *me*.

The message was this:

>A new strength . . .
>
>There are times in every life
>when we feel hurt or alone . . .
>But I believe that these times
>when we feel lost
>and all around us seems
>   to be falling apart
> are really bridges of growth.
>We struggle and try to recapture
>   the security of what was,
>   but almost in spite of ourselves . . .
>we emerge on the other side
> with a new understanding,
> a new awareness,
> a new strength.
>It is almost as though
> we must go through the pain
>   and the struggle
>   in order to grow
>and reach new heights.
>
>by: *Sue Mitchell. 1981.*
>*Copyright © Blue Mountain Arts, Inc.*
>*All rights reserved.*
>*Reprinted by permission of*
>*Blue Mountain Arts.*

My sister's special friend is now my special friend.

There are special sympathy cards for when parents, grandparents, or children die. After Andrea died, I noticed that most card stores did not have any sympathy cards for when siblings die!

SIB-A-THY® CARD INFORMATION FORM

The sibling relationship is very special. After sibling death, brothers and sisters deserve to receive special sympathy cards to help them celebrate and remember their special relationships.

Letters from a Friend authors, like *you,* have designed

SIB-A-THY® Cards.
SIB-A-THY® Cards are special sympathy cards which will be sold
under the copyright of:
© *2001 Erika Barber. All rights reserved.*

The cards are designed just for brothers and sisters whose siblings have died. Some of the money collected from the card sales may help siblings, like you, in many ways.

Use a blank page to design a SIB-A-THY® Card.

> Remember:
> There can be many different kinds of SIB-A-THY® Cards. In your design, you may write a special message and/or draw a picture.

Your Name: _____

Your Age: _____

Write a sentence about your sibling who died.
_____

This form, along with your card design, must be mailed with the SIB-A-THY® Card Consent Form. (The consent form is on the next page.) Your card design or portions of the design will not be processed without the completed consent form and information form.
SIB-A-THY® is a registered trademark.

SIB-A-THY® CARD CONSENT FORM

Your design or portions of your design will not be printed or sold without a completed and signed consent form and information form. The SIB-A-THY® Card Information Form is on the previous page.

You must be at least 18 years old to complete your own consent form. Card designers who are 17 years old or younger must have a parent or legal guardian complete the consent form.

Completed and signed consent forms may be sent along with your SIB-A-THY® Card design and information form to the address on the dedication page of this guide.

Use scissors to clip at dotted line. Mail in the consent form below.

- -

I, _____, am the card designer and am at least 18 years old, or I am the
     please print your name
parent or legal guardian of _____. I hereby give consent to
                             please print name of card designer
Erika Barber to print and sell the enclosed SIB-A-THY® Card design or portions of the design. I understand that the design or portions of the design may be printed as a card which may be sold to the general public. I also understand that the printed card may include information such as the card designer's name, age, city, state, country and other information (with the exception of phone numbers) for the purposes of the SIB-A-THY® Card Program.

Therefore, I hereby waive all rights on behalf of the card designer and his or her family to publicity and privacy as it relates to the SIB-A-THY® Card program. I hereby irrevocably grant a royalty-free assignment of copyright for all rights to the design of the SIB-A-THY® Card to Erika Barber. I hereby waive any moral rights on behalf of the card designer and his or her family to the design of the SIB-A-THY® Card.

I understand that a portion of the proceeds collected from the card sales may be utilized by Erika Barber to foster and enrich this program's philosophies and goals, and that I, the card designers and/or their families may not claim or collect proceeds acquired from the card sales. I understand that Erika Barber, her employees, successors, and assigns are not responsible and shall not be held liable in any way for specific outcomes or developments relating to the SIB-A-THY® Card Program. Erika Barber reserves the right to edit, revise or refuse any submitted SIB-A-THY® Card design.

I HAVE READ, I UNDERSTAND, AND I AGREE TO ALL OF THE ABOVE.

Signed _____
                        please sign your name

Your relationship to the card designer _____
(If you are completing this form, and you are also the SIB-A-THY® Card designer, you must submit proof that you are 18 years or older. For example, a photocopy of your driver's license or other identification which states your age.)

Date _____

Card Designer's City _____ State _____ Country _____

Card Designer's Phone Number (___) _____
                        for SIB-A-THY® Card files only

38 / LETTERS FROM A FRIEND

Design a sympathy card collage or picture with the sympathy cards you received after your brother or sister died.

> Ask an adult in your family if you may also use sympathy cards that your family received for this activity.

Glue or tape your sympathy card design on this paper. You may also use scissors and clip special words or illustrations from the cards for your collage or picture.

Visiting My Sibling's Body

VISITING THE CEMETERY

My sister's body was buried in the ground under a huge evergreen tree and near a twisting road inside a cemetery.

For months after Andrea died, I did not like going to the cemetery to see her grave. Mostly, I didn't like going, because I had to go with my parents. I stood beside my mother and father and watched them as they cried. I listened to them as they talked to Andrea's headstone and as they shared, with me, their memories of my sister. I felt sad watching and listening to them. I thought I had to be emotionally strong for both my parents, so I did not cry.

When I was able to drive a car by myself, I wanted to see Andrea's grave. I went to the cemetery alone and stood or sat near the marbled headstone. Sometimes, I stayed there for hours. I cried, I yelled, and I talked to my sister about things which we used to talk about in her bedroom, late at night.

On summer days, the cemetery was peaceful. I liked to sit on the mossy grass and pull weeds from Andrea's grave. Deer sometimes hid behind the trees which were scattered around the cemetery, and geese drank water from a large cement fountain. Bumble-bees and butterflies sniffed the smells from the flowers which my mother had potted around the grave. Squirrels harvested nuts among the pine needles.

There was so much life in the cemetery!

I still visit the cemetery, sometimes. I still believe Andrea's body is buried beneath that evergreen. Everyday, I think about Andrea, and every time I think about her, I feel a warm, special place inside me. I believe that is where Andrea's memory really is, and I can visit that place, anytime.

While a person is alive, he or she may decide what will happen to his or her body after death. Some people decide to have their bodies buried in the ground, inside cemeteries or in other special places. Sometimes, a person's body may be placed inside a special building, called a mausoleum. After death, a body may also be cremated or made into ashes. The ashes may be given to the dead person's family. Some people choose to have their bodies donated to medical or educational programs after death. Parts of their bodies may be donated to help sick or injured people become healthy.

MY SIBLING'S BODY

While your sibling was alive, did he or she decide what would happen to his or her body after death? Share:

Since your brother or sister died, where is your sibling's body? Draw a picture of the special place.

If you do not know, draw a picture of the place you think your sibling's body is.
(It may be helpful to share your drawing with an adult you trust.)

SHARE YOUR FEELINGS ABOUT VISITING THE LOCATION OF YOUR BROTHER OR SISTER'S BODY

You may write a poem or a story, or just describe your feelings.

Sometimes, family and friends decorate the location of a dead person's body. Decorating is a special way of remembering the person who died.

After your brother or sister's death, there are many ways you may decorate the location of your sibling's body:

Ask an adult you trust to help you with your decorations.

- make, then post, a picture or photo collage;
- plant a seed;
- play a special song or read a special story, poem or letter at the location of your sibling's body. Then, post the lyrics, story, poem or letter there;
- make, then mount, a wreath;
- make, then display, decorations for different holidays or for the seasons.

> Remember:
> If you are unable to visit the location of your sibling's body, choose a special place where you can remember your brother or sister who has died. You may be able to decorate that special place, too.

Sometimes, after a death, the dead person's name, birthday and the day he or she died are printed on a sign or on a headstone. A headstone is a special marker which is placed in the ground where a dead person is buried. If the letters on the sign or headstone are bumpy, a copy print of the sign or headstone can be made.

If there is a sign or headstone near the location of your sibling's body, try making a print. Place this piece of paper over the letters on the sign or headstone. Then, rub a pencil or crayon over the letters until you can see the letters appear on this paper.

A Print of My Sibling's Sign or Headstone

Returning To School

> Soon after your brother or sister's death, complete this activity with an adult in your family. Then, give this form to your teacher or choose an adult you trust to give this form to your teacher.

Date _____

Dear _____,
              name of teacher

I want you to know that my sibling _____
                                                       name of sibling who died

died on _____.
                                date sibling died

Death services are scheduled for _____
                                         dates and times of death services

at _____.
                              locations of death services

Please share the following information with my classmates before I return to school:
_____
_____.

Please do not share the following information with my classmates:
_____
_____.

I will not be in school during: _____.
                                       dates and times you plan to be absent

I plan to return to school on: _____.
                                     date and time you plan on returning to school

Homework assignments may be given to: _____.
                                             name of person responsible for getting your homework

The best time to speak with me or my family is _____.
                                             days and times you or your family will be available

For more information, please contact: _____.
                                        name of designated person and person's phone number

Thank you.
Sincerely,

_____
                your name

When you first return to school after your brother or sister's death, you may feel afraid, nervous, even excited. For awhile, concentrating during class or doing homework may seem difficult. Going back to school is important and may help you adjust to living your life since your brother or sister died. There may be times during the school day when you want to cry or be alone. Speak with your teacher if you want to leave the classroom for awhile, BUT if you continue crying for several days or leaving class often for emotional reasons, speak with a support person or your school counselor.

Planning your school schedule may help you cope with your return to school after your brother or sister's death.

Use the blank schedule or blank calendar at the end of this guide.

SCHOOL SUPPORT LIST

Since my brother or sister died, when I need emotional support at school, I can speak with:

Name   Phone Number   Office Number   Locker Number

My school counselors:

Teachers:

Friends:

Coaches:

Think about other people who may emotionally support you at school since your brother or sister died. Write their names on this list.

When you return to school after your brother or sister's death, there may be classmates, teachers and other school staff who may not know how to emotionally support you. Some people may be unsure of what to say to you or what to do for you.

Write a letter to the students and staff at your school. In your letter, describe how they can help you and what they can say or do to emotionally support you when you return to school after your sibling's death.

> Remember:
> You may ask a student or staff member you trust to share your letter with others before or when you return to school.

> Remember:
> People want to help you. It is not right to expect or misuse their help.

Many times there are no "correct" answers to questions about dying and death. Maybe that's why some teachers feel uncomfortable talking about dying and death.

EARNING THE GRADE

Grade each of your teachers and any other school staff members on how well he or she has emotionally supported you since your brother's or sister's death.

Assignment: *Emotionally Supporting Me Since My Sibling's Death*

Name	School Job	Grade Earned	Comments:
			(Describe your observations about each person or write about how each person could improve.)

A PLEDGE TO YOUR SIBLING

Since your brother or sister's death, design a school program which acknowledges or celebrates your sibling's life.

Acknowledgments and celebrations may include:

- a poem read to each class or written in the school newspaper;
- a class play or skit about your sibling's cause of death;
- a tree planted near the school, in memory of your brother or sister.

Ask a school staff member you trust to help you design a program or an activity to acknowledge or celebrate your brother or sister's life.

Use this page to design your program.

MY RELIGION AND MY GOD

MY RELIGION

My parents taught me about my god when I was a little girl. They taught me that my god knew when I did good things and when I did bad things. My god acted fairly. My god rewarded people who did good things and punished people who did bad things.

I learned about prayer. Praying was a way to talk to my god. In a prayer, I could also ask my god for things I wanted.

In Catholic religion class, I learned about souls. I learned that every person has a soul inside him or her. People with "good souls" do good things; people with "bad souls" do bad things. After a person's body died, I learned that a "good soul" goes to "Heaven" to be with my god, but a "bad soul" goes to a terrible place called "Hell."

After Andrea died, I felt very confused and angry with my god. Andrea's death seemed like a punishment for me. It seemed like a punishment I did not deserve. Andrea's death was not fair. I tried praying to my god. I asked my god to make my sister alive and healthy again, but that did not happen. It seemed that my god was ignoring me, so I decided to ignore my god. I stopped praying, and I stopped going to church.

My parents, religion teachers, and priests could not explain why Andrea was allowed to die. No one understood; no one could help me understand.

Sometimes, I'd look up toward the sky, where I believed Heaven was, and shout,

It's not fair! *You* do not act fairly!

> Remember:
> After your sibling's death, it is O.K. to feel angry with your god and with your religion. Anger is a part of grief!

Andrea did not die because of something bad she or I did. My god was not punishing my sister, my family or me when Andrea became ill or when she died.

I used to think my god made bad things happen to people who did bad things. Now, I believe bad things just happen.

A few months after Andrea's death, I started praying to my god again. I asked for emotional strength, for comfort and for peace instead of praying for things. Sometimes, I pray to Andrea. I tell Andrea about my feelings, my goals and about my life since she died. I believe, somehow, Andrea's soul and my god are near me. I believe my sister and my god listen to my prayers and maybe even share my feelings.

Bad things will probably happen again in my life, and I'll keep praying to my god and to Andrea. I'll keep believing that my god acts fairly and that my sister's soul is a good soul. Mostly, I'll know that I can live through the bad times, again. You can, too!

MY RELIGION

The name of my religion is _____.

Many people learn about death from religious lessons. What did you learn about death?

1.   4.

2.   5.

3.   6.

Since your sibling's death, has a religious person or thing helped you? How has the person or thing helped you?
WRITE:

What did your brother or sister believe happens to people after death?

What do you believe happened to your brother or sister after he or she died?
DRAW, using three crayons in your drawing.

Write a letter to your god. If you talk or pray to your god, write a prayer.

> Remember:
> You may share your letter or prayer with someone or just with yourself. Sharing your letter or prayer with a religious adult may help answer your questions about your sibling's death, about your religion, or help you feel better.

Use scissors and . . .

Clip words from a magazine which describe your feelings about your god or about your religion since your sibling's death. Glue or tape the words below.

MY SIBLING'S SOUL: ACTIVITIES

> Remember:
> When you have completed these activities, it may be helpful to share your drawings and your beliefs with an adult you trust.

Some people believe that every living thing has a soul. After a body dies, the soul does not die. If you believe your brother or sister has a soul, where is your sibling's soul since your brother or sister died? Draw a picture of the special place.

What do you believe your sibling's soul does?

1.

2.

3.

There are also people who believe that a dead person will live again in a different form, as a different person or as an animal. This belief is called "reincarnation."

If you believe in reincarnation, draw a picture of your brother or sister in his or her new living form, as a different person or as an animal.

Grief Feelings

Every feeling you feel about your sibling and about your sibling's death is important. Sharing your feelings is important, too. Sharing your feelings by writing, drawing, or talking about your sibling is a wonderful way to remember your sibling who died. You may also feel better after sharing your feelings.

> Remember:
> It is O.K. to talk about your sibling's *illness, injury, accident, murder, suicide,* or other cause of his or her death. It is also O.K. to say or to write these words.

Grieving is a healthy experience for many people after a death happens. During healthy grieving, a person learns to cope with a death and with the many changes which may happen after a death. The feelings a person feels after a death happens may be called "grief feelings." All of the grief feelings shared in this guide are O.K. for you to feel after your sibling's death. These feelings, and other feelings you may have, are part of healthy grieving.

> Remember:
> Your sibling relationship is special to you, so your grief feelings will also be special. People in your family, even your other siblings, may grieve differently than you do.

At different times in your life, you may feel confused or not understand how you feel since your sibling died. That is O.K., too. Grieving can be hard work—but *you can do it!*

> Remember:
> There is not a "right time" to start grieving your sibling's death, but starting is important!

Throughout your life, you may feel many of the grief feelings shared in this guide. You will probably have new understandings about your feelings as you grow older.

> Remember:
> There is not a "certain length of time" you are supposed to feel an emotion. Your grief feelings and how long you feel them are special to you!

YOU ARE A "SURVIVOR"!

After your sibling's death, you will be surviving every day of your life. You may feel better on some days than on others, even years after your sibling's death.

> Remember:
> The days you do not feel better are still part of healthy grieving.

Usually, people are called "survivors" after they have lived through terrible experiences, like tornadoes or storms at sea. The experience of a brother or a sister's death may seem even more terrible. *You d*eserve to be called a "survivor," because you have chosen to live your life while grieving your sibling's death.

Some people may believe that talking about their siblings or sharing their grief feelings about their siblings' death may cause other bad things to happen.

It won't.

Some people may not talk about their siblings or share their grief feelings about their siblings' death, because they or other people may cry or feel sad.

It is O.K. to cry and to feel sad. Sadness and crying are part of healthy grieving.

Some people may not talk about their siblings or share their grief feelings about their siblings' death, because they believe their grief feelings will "go away" without talking or sharing.

Some people are able to ignore their grief feelings, but their feelings will not "go away." Ignored feelings may cause other problems in your life, even years after your sibling's death. These problems may be even more difficult to work through than working through your grief is now.

There are many opportunities to share grief feelings in the next few sections. Choose the sections and activities to include in your book.

> Remember:
> If you feel too much of a certain emotion,
> share your grief feelings with an adult you trust.

Reminders:

> You don't need to be emotionally strong for anyone! Share your grief feelings, too.

> Sometimes, people who seem emotionally strong, or people who do not share their grief emotions, need the most help grieving!

> You are special. Your grief is different from anyone else's grief!

It may be helpful to read the pages about my sister's death before continuing in the guide. The pages are in the section titled "My Sibling's Death."

Denial

"MY SIBLING IS NOT DEAD!"

"Andrea died."

"NO!"

"NO!"

"NO!"

I thought, "My neighbor is lying! She misunderstood my father's message when he called from the hospital! My sister can't be dead!"

I screamed, "NO!"

My body fell to the floor.

"This isn't supposed to happen to me—not to my family!" I cried as I walked through the hospital emergency room doors.

In the examination room, I poked and pushed Andrea's body. I shook her arms and tried opening my sister's eyes. Andrea really was dead.

> I saw my sister's dead body.
> I read the sympathy cards which were sent to my family.
> I went to my sister's death services.

Still, sometimes, I pretended Andrea was alive and that her death did not really happen. Sometimes, I imagined that Andrea was still on her vacation in Europe.

> And, for awhile, I did not feel my emotional pain.

I went to school and studied four hours each day and earned all "A's" on my report card and really didn't think about Andrea at all.

> And, for awhile, I did not feel my emotional pain.

My friends took me out to movies, out to dinner, and out to parties and I was too busy to think about Andrea's death.

> And, for awhile, I did not feel my emotional pain.

Andrea's bed was neatly made. My sister's eyeglasses and her retainer were still on her nightstand. Headbands and hair brushes were still in her dresser drawer. "Andrea must be coming home soon," I pretended.

> And, for awhile, I did not feel my emotional pain.
> But, after awhile, I felt the emotional pain again.

When do you feel less emotional pain about your brother's or sister's death?

_____

_____.

    And, for awhile, I do not feel my emotional pain.

_____

_____.

    And, for awhile, I do not feel my emotional pain.

_____

_____.

    And, for awhile, I do not feel my emotional pain.

Do you ever think that your brother or sister is not dead?
Write about this thought:

> Remember:
> It may be helpful to share your thoughts with an adult you trust.

56 / LETTERS FROM A FRIEND

Since she died, I think I've seen . . .

>   Andrea on the television news.
>   My sister's face in magazine ads.
>   Andrea driving a car through town.

Since Andrea died, I've seen many strangers who look like my sister used to look. There are even some people whose voices sound like Andrea's voice used to sound. Each time I encounter these strangers, I am reminded that my sister really is dead. I am reminded of the sadness and confusion I felt the day Andrea died.

There are times, though, when I see strangers who remind me of Andrea, and I smile. I smile, because even though my sister is dead, many of her features are still alive in other people.

Since your sibling's death . . .
have you ever believed you saw or heard your brother or sister?

Share these experiences and your feelings about these experiences.

> Remember:
> It may be helpful to share this activity with an adult you trust.

When or where does your sibling's death become more real or believable?
WRITE:

Anger

You may feel or have felt angry about your sibling's death for many reasons.

Express your anger in a poem. Use this page to create your own poem or to share your thoughts about a poem which was already written. Poems do not always rhyme.

> Remember:
> You may share your poem with someone you trust or just with yourself.

Write the poem here:

Written by: _____

When you feel angry, how do you express it?

> Remember:
> Ignoring your anger will not make it go away.

Some people express their anger by slamming doors, swearing, or breaking things. Sometimes a person may shout at people or things with which he or she does not feel angry! Behavior like this is called *displacement*. All feelings may be displaced sometimes, but it may be especially harmful to displace anger!

Some people do not express their anger at all. Unexpressed feelings, especially unexpressed anger, may also be harmful.

SCREAM THERAPY!

Find a special place where no one will be disturbed when you do this activity.
(I did this activity in my basement when no one was at home. Sometimes I screamed into a pillow.)

Why have you felt angry about your brother's or sister's death? Think about the reasons for your anger. Then . . . as loudly as you can . . .

SCREAM!!!   YELL!!!   SHOUT!!!

There are many other ways to express your anger about your sibling's death without hurting someone or damaging something. What are some "other ways"?

Share your ideas:

WANTED: FOR MY SIBLING'S DEATH

Who or what caused your brother or sister to die? Place the photo or draw a picture of the person or thing. Share this activity with an adult you trust.

Inside this imaginary courtroom . . .

Draw a picture of yourself. You are the judge.
Draw a picture of the person or thing responsible for your brother or sister's death.
Draw pictures of any other people or things in this imaginary court room.

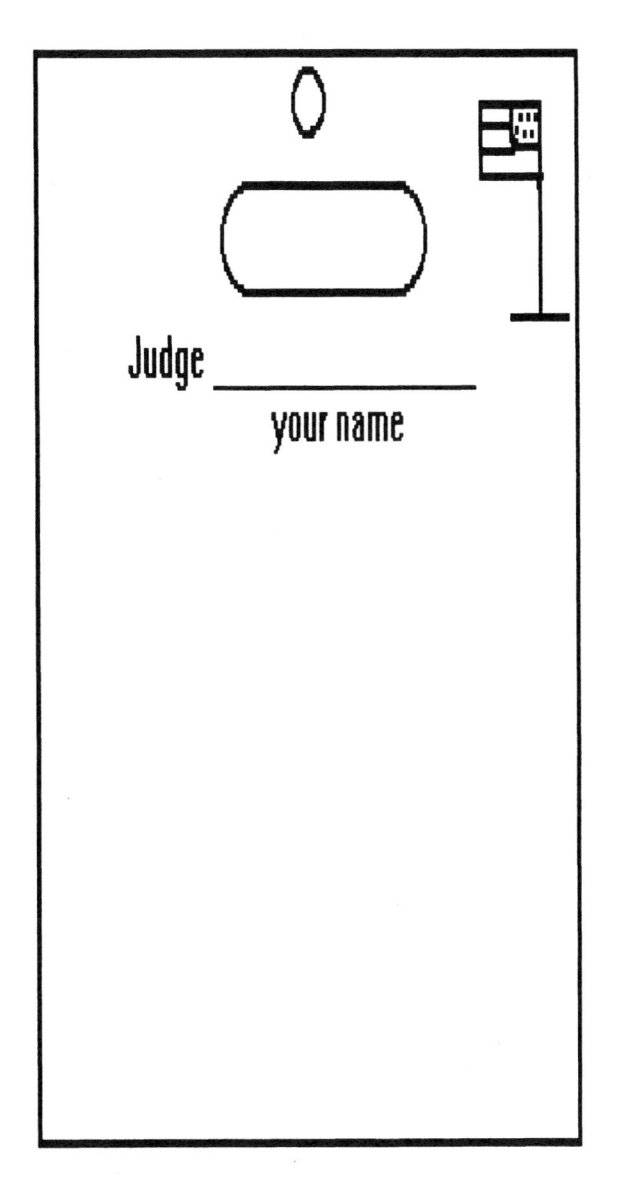

Judge _____
your name

What punishment will you give the person or thing?

_____
_____
_____
_____

Remember:
It may be helpful to share this activity with an adult you trust.

You may feel or have felt angry about your brother or sister's death for many reasons. With whom or what do you feel or have you felt angry? Write a letter to the person or thing about your anger.

If you displaced your anger, and expressed anger toward someone or something with which you *did not feel angry,* write to this person or thing. (You may learn more about "displaced feelings" at the beginning of this section.)

> Remember:
> You may share your letter with someone you trust or just with yourself.

When do you feel or have you felt most angry about your brother's or sister's death? Use this page to draw a picture or write about your anger.

When you have finished this activity, tear this page from the guide and RIP IT UP!!!

Glue or tape the pieces on the next page.

Think about a group or an organization which relates to your sibling's death in some way. Some groups and organizations are:

- cancer awareness groups—if your sibling died because of his or her cancer
- groups against driving under the influence of alcohol or drugs—if your sibling's death was related to such a situation
- Representatives and Senators of your state (They have the power to make and change laws)
- Other Political Leaders

You may get addresses for special groups and organizations from the phone book or from a resource person or book.

Use a separate page of paper to write a letter to the group or organization you choose.

In your letter, share your thoughts, feelings and ideas about:

- The improvements or changes which the group or organization could make, so that less people would die the way your sibling died.
- How the group or organization could help siblings whose brothers and sisters are dying or after their brothers or sisters have died, the way your sibling died.

> Remember:
> You do not need to mail your letter. Just writing may help you feel better.

TREASURES

A few months after my sister's death, my mother still had all of Andrea's belongings. I felt angry with my mother because I didn't want to see anything which used to belong to my sister.

"Andrea won't need any of her things ever again!" I yelled at my mom. I wanted to throw away my sister's:

- violin
- clothes
- jewelry box
- eyeglasses and contact lenses
- school books
- make-up
- photo albums

Many years later, I understood that I never actually felt angry with my mother because she kept my sister's belongings. I felt angry with *my sister* because she died. I felt anger because whenever I saw something which used to belong to Andrea, I was reminded of her death.

I still have a few things which my sister gave me. I call these things my "treasures." I have:

- the porcelain heart necklace, a present she let me open before Christmas Day, one year;
- the perfume she left for me, before she died;
- the black leather pants she bought for me, when she was vacationing in Europe.

Photographs of Andrea are very special to me now, too. I don't feel anger anymore when I see photos of my sister. I have two black and white photographs of Andrea in my wallet. When I look at the photos, I notice the similarities between my sister and me, and I feel happy about them. Even though I am a different person than my sister was, I believe the similarities are another way Andrea's memory is always with me.

Years after my sister's death, my mother led me into the basement of her new house. We walked past the laundry room and stopped beside a small wooden cabinet. My mother reached her frail, bony hands into the cabinet, then pulled a cardboard box onto the tile floor. She lifted the box top. The box was filled with photo albums. Each album had many photographs of Andrea and me.

There were photos of me when I was a baby . . .
photos of Andrea, taken on her first day of school
and on the day she graduated from high school.

The air smelled of damp basement and musty album pages. While sitting on the cold tile floor and breathing the musty smells, Mom and I looked at photos and shared our memories:

"Mom, that's when Andrea took me to the zoo!"   "I remember."

"Look, Mom! I found the Easter basket that year again."   "Actually, Erika, Andrea always let you find it!"

"Remember Burford, Mom?"   "You girls loved that guinea pig! That photo was taken after he won the contest for 'Longest-haired animal'."

Mom and I laughed as we shared our memories. We cried together a little, too. Before she put the box top back on, Mom said, "Take the photos you want. These albums really belong with you, now. Cherish them, Erika."   I am, Mom.

1.

2.

3.

4.

5.

    Make a list of the "treasures," or things you want to keep, as memories of your brother or sister who died.

> Remember:
> You may ask an adult you trust to help you or to complete this activity for you, if you do not feel comfortable or ready to do it.

    You may also get a box or chest. Inside the box or chest, place photos of your brother or sister who died, sympathy cards you received after your sibling's death, and other special treasures which belonged to your sibling or which your brother or sister gave to you before he or she died.

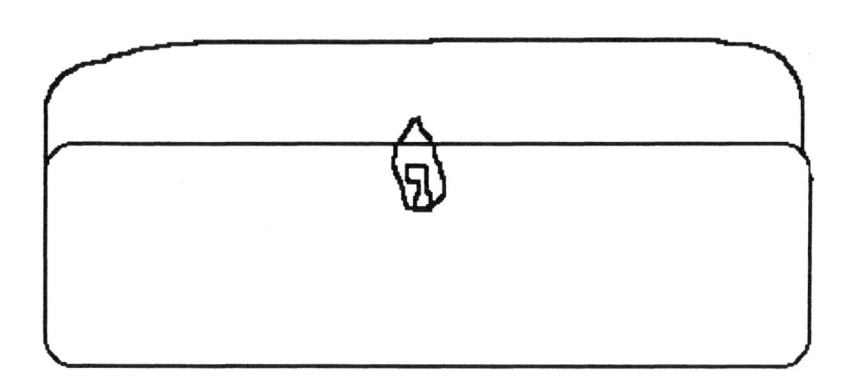

Sadness

I feel *so* sad!

After my sister died, I felt sad for a very long time. I had felt sad before, during my life, like when I lost my homework and when my pet rabbit died, but this sadness was different, somehow.

This sadness seemed powerful, as if I would never feel any other emotion, except sadness, for the rest of my life.

I felt sadness inside my body. My head seemed heavy on my shoulders. Sometimes, my head seemed to tingle or buzz. I couldn't think about anything. My legs and arms seemed weak. I didn't want to move or talk or feel.

For a long time after Andrea's death, there seemed to be a huge empty space inside my body. There were many empty spaces after my sister died: Andrea's chair at the dinner table, my sister's empty space in the toothbrush holder, my sibling relationship in my life.

My chest seemed tight, and my heart seemed heavy. I imagined all the reasons for my sadness were written inside my heart. I wished I could see inside my heart, to see these reasons and to help me express my sadness about Andrea's death. Maybe then, my heart would seem lighter, and the empty spaces would seem full again.

I have no more siblings.
My children will never meet their Aunt Andrea.
I couldn't save my sister's life.
I won't get advice from Andrea anymore.
Andrea will never be the teacher she wanted to be.
My family will never be the same.

Why have you felt sad about your sibling's death?

Write about the reasons for your sadness inside the heart.

> Remember:
> There may be many times throughout your life when you feel sad about your sibling's death. Soon, you may be able to think about your brother or sister and feel less sadness. Also, remember: it is O.K. to cry.

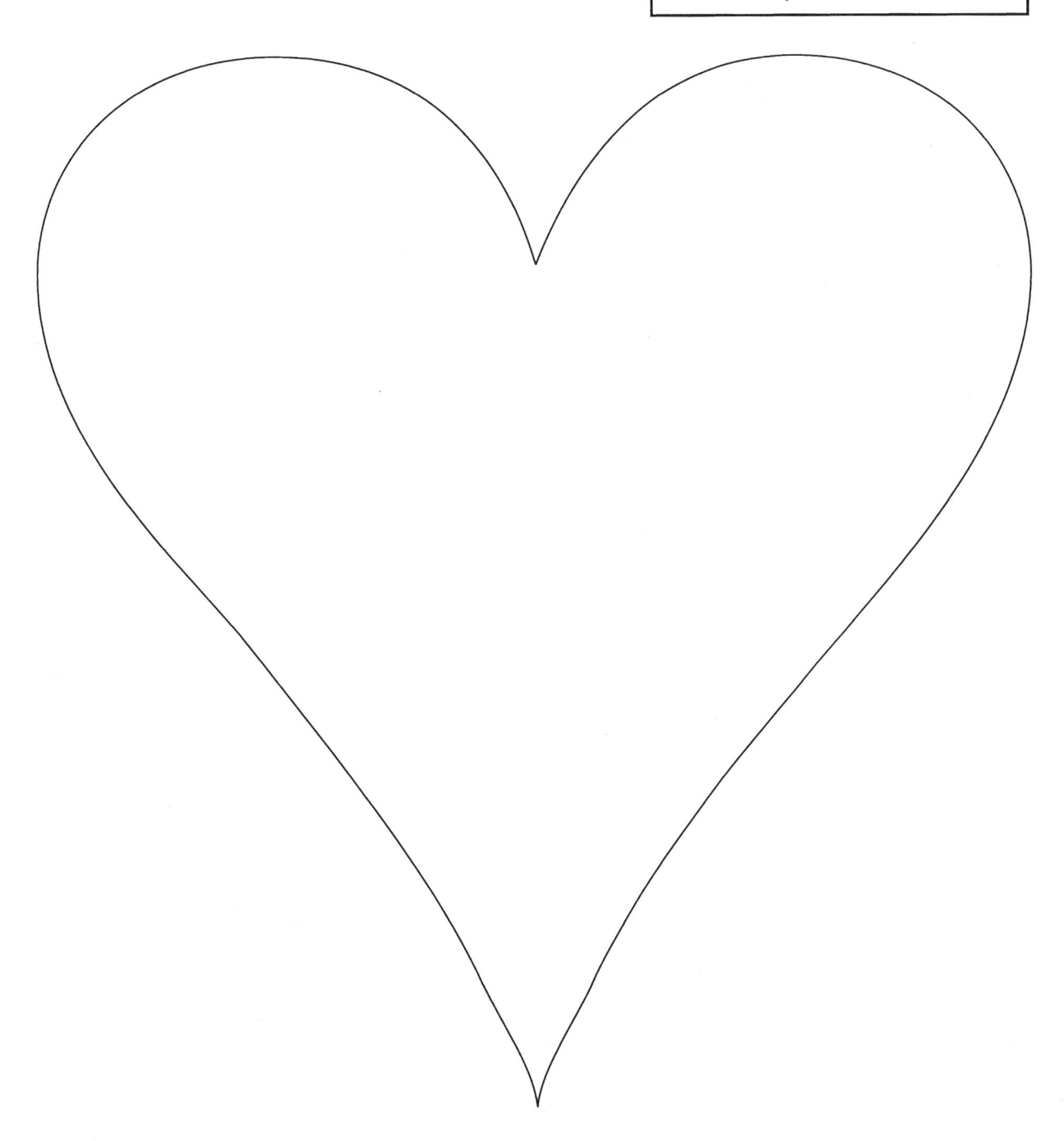

Think about the habits or things your brother or sister did which annoyed you. Do you miss some of these things since your brother or sister died?

Write a letter to your sibling about these things you miss.

Dear _____ ,

> Remember:
> You may share your letter with someone you trust or just with yourself.

SONG OF SADNESS

As a teenager, Andrea loved to play and to listen to all kinds of music. She played her violin, and, for hours, she listened to and tape recorded "new wave" and "punk rock" music. Many times, Andrea hummed or created new words to songs. Andrea even turned on the radio to help her sleep.

Since she died, I've often thought about Andrea while listening to song lyrics. The singers seemed to express my grief feelings, and I felt comforted knowing that I wasn't the only person who had ever felt grief emotions.

One song was on the radio, just weeks after Andrea died. Since then, I have never heard another song like it. I bought a record of the song, and I still listen to it when I'm feeling sad and missing Andrea in my life.

Christopher Cross is the singer, and the song is called,

"Think of Laura."

These are the lyrics:

Every once in a while I'd see her smile
And she'd turn my day around
A girl with those eyes
Could stare through the lies
And see what your heart was saying

Think of Laura but laugh don't cry
I know she'd want it that way
When you think of Laura laugh don't cry
I know she'd want it that way

A friend of a friend
A friend to the end
That's the kind of girl she was
Taken away so young
Taken away without a warning

I know you and you're here
In every day we live
I know her and she's here
I can feel her when I sing

Hey Laura, where are you now
Are you far away from here
I don't think so
I think you're here
Taking our tears away

© 1983 BMG Songs, Inc. (ASCAP)
Warner Brother Records, Inc. for the United States
All rights reserved. Used by permission.
Writer: Christopher Cross
Title: Think of Laura

Many times, when I feel sad about Andrea's death, I cry. Usually, my body seems weak after I cry, but I do feel better.

After my sister died, I cried a lot. Sometimes, I cried with my parents, but most times, I cried when I was alone. When I grew older, I liked to go to Andrea's grave and cry. I stayed at the cemetery and cried for hours. Afterwards I felt relaxed and emotionally strong enough to survive another day.

70 / LETTERS FROM A FRIEND

Express the sadness you are feeling or have felt about your sibling's death in a song or poem. Use this page to create your own song or poem or to share your thoughts about a song or poem which was already written.

Name of song or poem: _____

Performed by: _____

Written by: _____

Have you ever wanted to die to be with your brother or sister? Have you wanted to die to stop feeling grief emotions?

> Remember:
> It is O.K. to want your brother or sister to be alive again.
> It is O.K. to want to be with your brother or sister and to want to stop feeling grief emotions . . .
> BUT,
> if you ever want to die,
> TELL AN ADULT YOU TRUST!!!
>
> **You and your life are important.**

It's Not Fair

MY "IT'S NOT FAIR!" FEELING

The **"It's Not Fair!"** feeling is sometimes called "jealousy" or "envy." People who feel very jealous may be described as "green with envy."

<u>The Garden of Envy</u>

In the garden of envy
I sat all alone,
Watching others play
With siblings of their own.

    And slowly it grew, the vine of ivy,
    Forming a green wall between them and me.

While Mom and Dad cried,
And in space they would stare,
Did anyone notice that I was still there?

Who will be at class elections
If I'm voted to win?
What college forms do I need to send in?

    And slowly it grew, the vine of ivy,
    Forming a green wall between them and me.

And who will help me,
When I'm missing her too?
Everyone's on their own,
By themselves, feeling "blue."

While kids my age wonder
Which new outfits to buy,
I wonder, "Why do kids my age
And younger die?"

    And slowly it grew, the vine of ivy,
    Forming a green wall between them and me.

There are some things in life
I think no one should have to do,
Like survive the death of a young sibling,
My Andrea, you . . .

Our sibling competition needs finally to end.
I still call you my sister; I still call you my friend.
It's not fair to compare us, to keep her room a "shrine."
She had her life, and I still have mine.

Yet, there are times, even now, when I feel envious of the others,
Those who still have their sisters and brothers.
And it is during these times, when the envy seems to grow stronger,
And it seems that the ivy grows longer and longer,
Until, soon, I think the ivy has separated me,
Leaving me feeling alone, and "green with envy."

YOUR "GARDEN OF ENVY"

What do you think is or was unfair about or since your sibling's death? Write about your thoughts on each paper "leaf of ivy."

> Share this activity with an adult you trust.

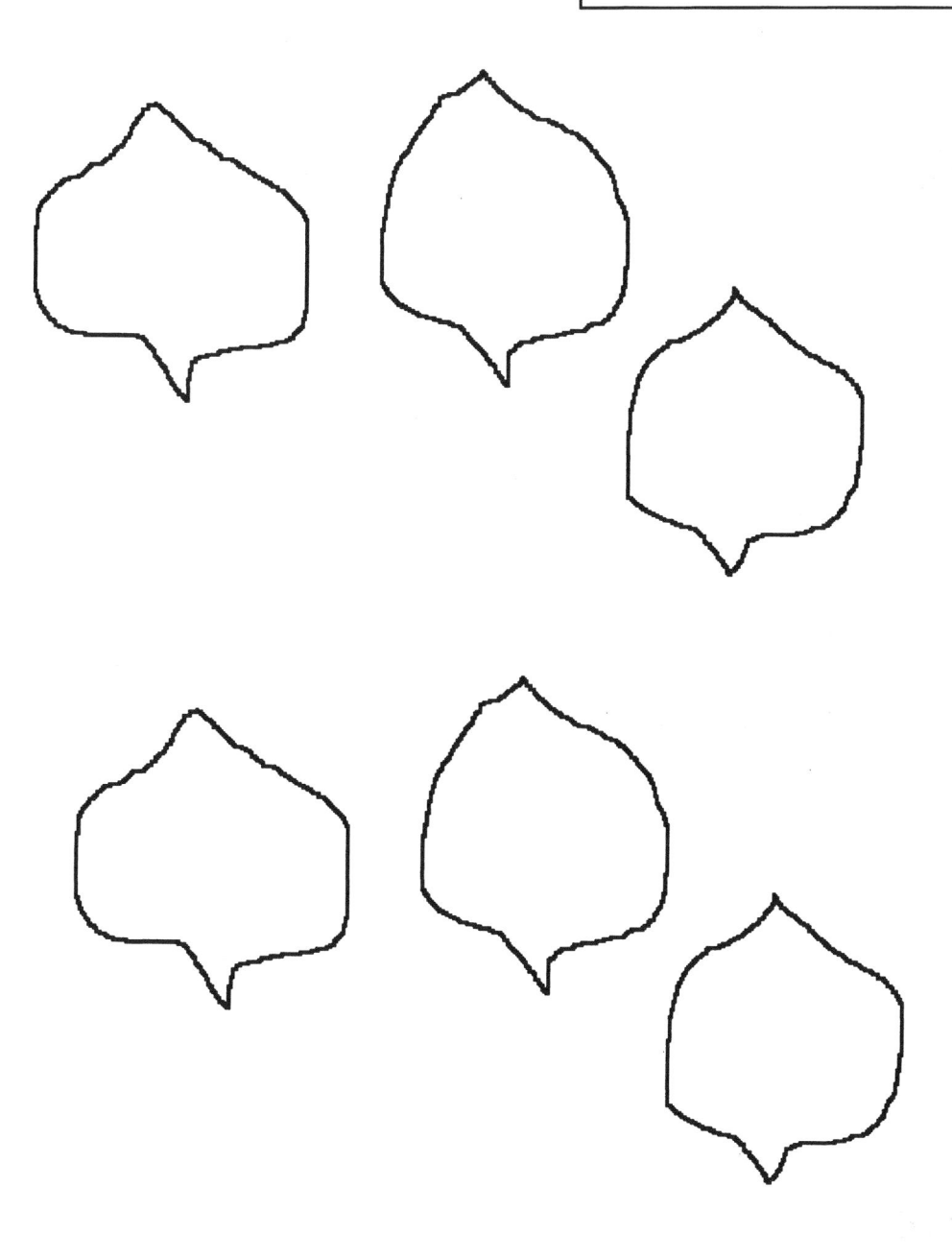

Guilt/If I Had Only

GUILT OR THE "IF I HAD ONLY" FEELING

Sometimes, people feel angry with themselves. This feeling is called "guilt." If the guilt feeling is not shared, people may continue to feel angry with themselves.

One winter night, years after my sister's death, I locked the bathroom door. I sat on the vanity and stared at my face in the mirror. I didn't like the person staring back at me.

I felt angry with the person . . . with *myself!*

I was finally ready to share the reasons for my guilt, and I chose to share them with myself. I thought about the December day when Andrea died. I imagined myself being 15 years old again. I said to my reflection,

"I feel angry with you, because you:

> said and did nasty things to Andrea while she was alive!"

> always tried to be more beautiful, smarter, or more loved than Andrea, even after she died!"

> didn't tell Andrea 'I love you' more while she was alive."

> didn't stop Andrea's death from happening."

> lived."

Share this activity with an adult you trust.

MIRROR TALKING

Get a mirror and find a quiet place to do this activity.

Since your sibling's death, why do you feel or have you felt angry with yourself?
Look at your reflection in the mirror. Then, share the reasons for your guilt with *yourself.*

I feel or felt angry with myself, because . . . (Write your responses inside the frames below.)

Remember:
Most brothers and sisters argue and say or think nasty about each other.
Your sibling did not die because of something you said, thought or wished.

Remember:
You can not change anything which has already happened. You can practice forgiving yourself for your past behavior and learn to change your future behavior!

76 / LETTERS FROM A FRIEND

Write about some "good" or positive things you have done:

With Or For Your Brother Or Sister While Your Sibling Was Alive

Since Your Sibling's Death

> Remember:
> You did what you were able to do at that particular time in your life!

NICE AND NASTY

While she was alive, Andrea and I did many "nice" things for each other. We also did many "nasty" things *to* each other!

Here are some "nice and nasties":

Andrea		Erika (me)	
Nice	Nasty	Nice	Nasty
Cooked meals for me	Locked me out of my room	Didn't tell my parents she tried to smoke a cigarette	Spied on her when she kissed her boyfriend
Let me jump on the bed when she baby-sat for me	Wrestled me on the living room carpet until my face turned blue	Visited her while she was hospitalized	Told her Mom and Dad wished she was more like me (when they hadn't)
Braided my hair	Called me "pest," "stupid," and "brat" during our arguments	Told her she looked pretty when she was getting ready for a date	Called her "loser," "idiot," and "dip" during our arguments
Told me which balloon had the penny prize in it at my friend's eighth birthday party	Threw oatmeal at my face, just because I dared her to do it	Bought five packs of chewy candies she was selling for her German club's fund-raiser (even though I hated chewy candies!)	Told her "I wish you were dead!" during our arguments

Think about your brother or sister who died. It may be difficult, at first, to remember "nice" or "nasty" things that you and your sibling did for or to each other while your brother or sister was alive. Under the columns below, write about the "nice and nasties" you and your sibling shared.

> Remember:
> Your brother or sister was not a perfect person. You are not a perfect person. Most siblings do "nice and nasty" things for and to each other.

Your Brother Or Sister		You	
Nice	Nasty	Nice	Nasty

If you could see "guilt," how do you think it would look?

DRAW

Describe each part of your drawing.

Afraid

SAFE PLACE

Sometimes, when I feel afraid, I visit a special place. In that place:

- the sun is always bright
- the sky is always blue
- there are vast beaches of white, smooth sand

In that place, blue waves gently roll over each other toward the shoreline. Near the shore, the waves finally spread outward, over the sandy tips of seashells. The blue, cool water drifts back to the ocean the same way, every time: over the tops of slippery moss-covered pebbles.

Besides the sound of muted waves rolling onto the shore, the beach area is quiet, and I feel comfortable there. Up on the bank, there are soft, green grasses. That is where the cave is hidden. No one, besides me, has ever seen the cave or the beach. No one has found that special, safe place—except me.

I can be alone on my beach. The cave is mine, too. In my special place, there is no pain, no fear, no worry.

I only wish my special place was real.

The beach and cave are inside me—inside my imagination. It is the safe place away from all my emotional pain, my fears, and my worries I have felt and had since my sister's death.

I discovered my special place on a cold November morning during a visit with a counselor. My counselor told me to close my eyes and think about a place where I felt safe . . . where I could stop thinking about Andrea's death for awhile . . . where I didn't have to worry about homework or parents—or anything.

Sometimes, now, it is difficult to think about my safe place without my counselor's help. Then, I go to a quiet room and close my eyes. Soon after, I can imagine the sun shining on my beach and the soothing waves on my shoreline. I think about the secret opening to my safe cave.

Since Andrea's death, I have visited my special place often. I've walked many imaginary miles in the moist white beach sand. Each time I visit, I discover the beauty of my special place:

- my beach can never be polluted with other people's garbage
- my green banks can never be destroyed for buildings or houses or streets
- my sea life can never become extinct

My special safe place will always belong to me.

Visiting my special place also helped me to better understand my fears about my sister's death.

My Fears	To Feel Less Afraid, I Can
I may get "severe depression" and die like my sister.	Share my fear with an adult who understands "severe depression." Learn the facts about the illness.
Other people I care about will die soon.	Share my fear with the people I care about. Learn about what would happen to me and to my life if they did die.
Becoming 20 years old (the age Andrea was when she died).	Ask my family and friends for emotional support when I become 20 years old. Share my fear, but still celebrate my 20th birthday!
The changes happening in my family since Andrea died.	Share my fear with Mom and Dad. Learn about the possible changes that may happen in my life.
Talking about Andrea, because someone may feel angry or cry if I do.	Share my memories of Andrea and my feelings with people I trust. It is O.K. and important to remember my sister. Feeling anger and crying are part of grieving.

You may feel or have felt afraid about or since your sibling's death.

Imagine a place where you can feel comfortable and safe. In your special place, you have no fears or worries.

> Remember:
> You can visit your special place anytime. You can feel safe again. What happened to your brother or sister probably does not happen to most children and teenagers. Share your fears with an adult you trust.

Draw a picture of your special place.

You may better understand your fears, too, after visiting your special place.

Write About:

My Fears

To Feel Less Afraid, I Can

> Remember:
> Sometimes, planning your daily schedule may help you feel less afraid and more in control of your life. Use the blank calendar or blank schedule at the end of this guide.

THE FEAR OF FORGETTING

Andrea and I shared 15-1/2 years together. I don't remember some of the times we shared, because I was a baby or a young child during many of those years. Yet, there are other events I shared with my sister when I was older, and I still can't seem to remember many of those experiences. Sometimes, I feel afraid that I'm forgetting those special times . . . that I'm forgetting Andrea.

Maybe, not remembering things about my sister or about Andrea's life is a way I am trying to forget the emotional pain I felt after Andrea's death. Even though I believe Andrea will always be part of my spiritual self, I don't ever want to forget that I once had a sister who was a physical part of my life.

Whenever I feel afraid of forgetting the special times my sister and I shared, or the special person Andrea was, I practice "room visiting."

During room visiting, I imagine or go to each room of the house in which Andrea and I lived together. Then I think about the special experiences Andrea and I shared in each room.

Memories in . . .

The Kitchen

- During dinner one night, Andrea bit into a cherry tomato. The seeds burst out from its side and sprayed across my face!

- Andrea slurped mashed potatoes and creamed corn through a straw. She had gotten her new braces the same day and her teeth felt sore!

- Andrea and I secretly fed our liver sausage sandwiches to our dog, who was beneath the kitchen table!

The Family Room

- Andrea and I snuggled on the couch and watched horror movies on Friday nights.

- Andrea pulled the corner of my pajama top from my mouth as I danced around the family room, and my loose tooth fell out!

- Andrea and I posed for Halloween photos: she was dressed as an exotic dancer, I as a doctor, and our dog as a ballerina!

Andrea's Bedroom

- Andrea and I locked her door, sat on her big bed, and talked loudly so that we wouldn't hear our parents arguing in the next room.

- During one of our arguments, I pushed Andrea off her bed and she sat on me until I cried.

- I sat on Andrea's bed while she braided my hair for six hours! When she was finished, I had 22 small braids and we both had sore butts!

ROOM VISITING

1. Imagine or go to the rooms or other special places you shared with your brother or sister who died.
2. Think about the experiences which happened in each place.
3. Write about your memories of your brother or sister.

Place: _____

Place: _____

Place: _____

Sometimes, speaking to other people who knew your brother or sister may help you recall special memories about your sibling who died.

Interview three people who knew your brother or sister. Ask them to share their memories about events or special times *you* shared with your sibling or just memories about your brother or sister.

What did you learn about your sibling relationship or about your brother or sister from the interviews?
WRITE:

VISITING THE PLACE MY SIBLING DIED

Visiting the place your sibling died may help you feel less afraid, help you understand many of your feelings, and help you remember special things about your brother or sister.

When you are emotionally ready, visit the place your brother or sister died. If you are unable to visit, imagine the place your sibling died.

Then . . . share your feelings and memories about the place and about your brother or sister.

> Remember:
> You may ask an adult you trust to help you complete this activity.

Has anything positive happened at or near the place since your sibling's death? Share:

FEELING LESS AFRAID

Sometimes, after traumatic experiences, people may feel *less* afraid of their fears. Since the traumatic event happened, a person may have learned about his or her fears or have new beliefs about his or her life.

Since your sibling died, do you feel less afraid about any of your fears? Share:

Some people believe that confronting their fears and having more experiences with their fears are healthy ways to feel less afraid. For example, people who feel afraid of snakes may practice watching, touching or holding snakes until they feel less afraid of them. Since your sibling's death, experiencing some of your fears may help you feel less afraid, too.

> Ask an adult you trust to help you with this activity.

Fear of:	Practice Experiences (After Your Sibling's Death):
Hospitals	Visit with the medical staff, visit a patient you know, volunteer in a hospital program
Funeral Homes	Visit the funeral home when no death services are planned or schedule to meet with the funeral home director

Share your fears. Then, share experiences to help you feel less afraid.

Fear of: Practice Experiences:

Joy/Happiness

One of the most important and special feelings you may feel since your sibling's death is joy or happiness.

You probably won't or didn't feel joyful or happy soon after your sibling's death, but it is important to remember that it is O.K. and healthy to feel joyful and happy again.

The day my sister died, one of my uncles told a joke about our dinner.

He said, "Looks like the chicken had a bad day, too."

I felt guilt because I laughed when my uncle told that joke. I didn't realize that it was O.K. to laugh and smile the same day Andrea died. Laughing and smiling did not mean I had forgotten about Andrea's death. It did not mean that I felt happy my sister died. Laughing and smiling were reminders that I was still alive. They were reminders that I could still feel joy and happiness, besides feeling all my grief emotions.

Since my sister's death, I feel joyful and happy about many things:

- My parents are healthy and feel happy.
- I have many friends.
- I have two furry and cuddly rabbits.
- I try helping other people, everyday.
- I am writing this guide for *you!*

When have you felt joyful or happy since your brother or sister's death? Write about the reasons for your joy or happiness in the frames below.

90 / LETTERS FROM A FRIEND

While Andrea was alive, there were many times I felt joyful and happy about my sister. Since she died, I think about these times:

> when Andrea danced with our dog across the living room floor

> when Andrea asked me to go to a movie with her and her friends

> when Andrea dressed in my father's pajamas

> when Andrea accidentally squirted toothpaste across the bathroom

> when Andrea taught me how to drive my dad's car (and didn't tell him I drove it)

While your sibling was alive, when did you feel joyful or happy about your brother or sister? Write about your memories in the frames below.

The Game of Survival

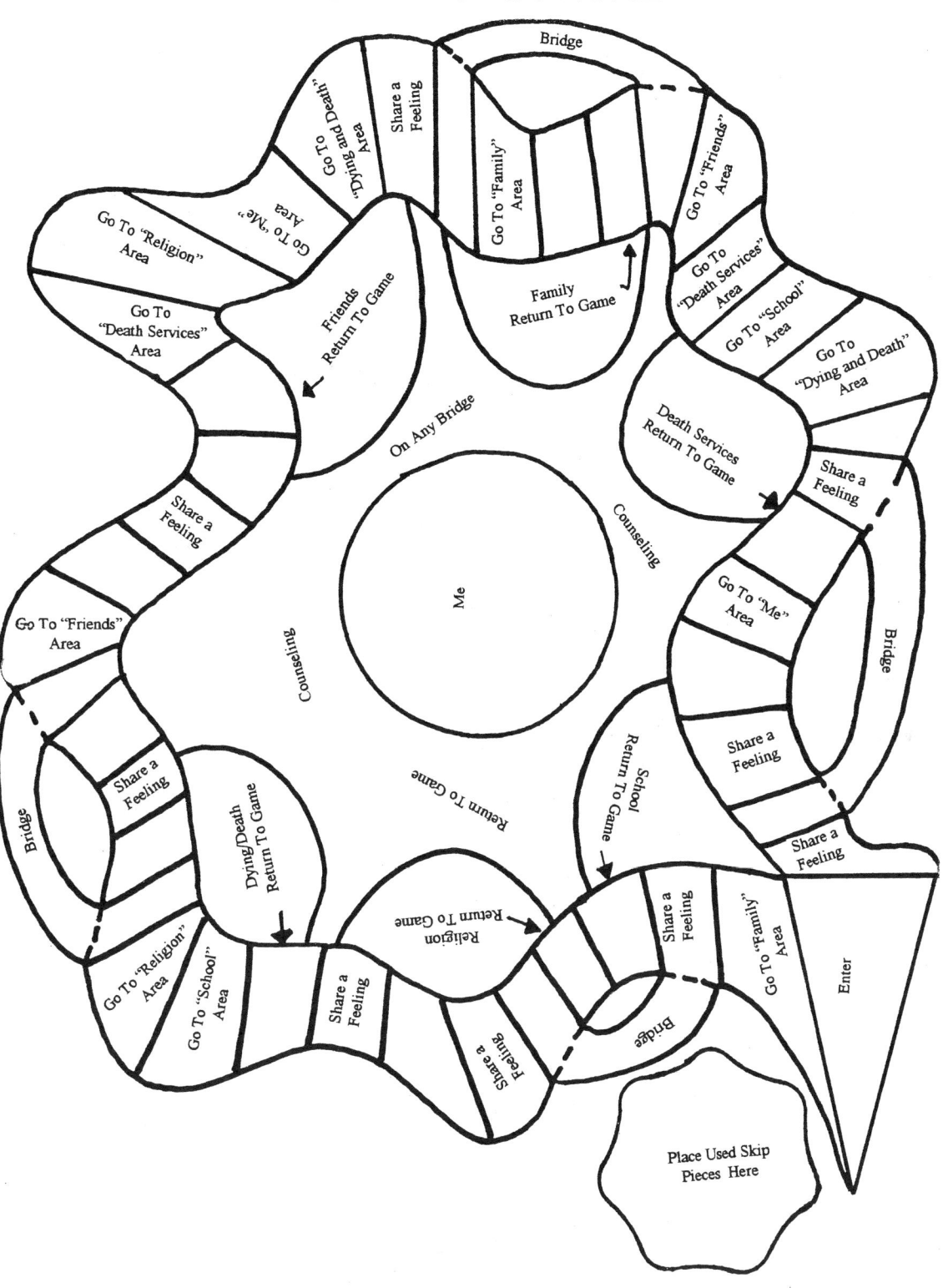

DIRECTIONS

This game may be played by 2 to 6 players.
The game is especially for players who knew your sibling when your brother or sister was alive.

You will need:
>scissors
>pencils or pens
>blank pieces of paper
>tape

Preparation:

1. Use scissors to clip out the "Playing Pieces," the "Skip Pieces," the "Feelings Cards"and the "Paper Dice." The game pieces, cards and "Paper Dice"are located on the next few pages.

2. Each player selects a "Playing Piece" and writes his or her name on it. Place "Playing Pieces" on the "Enter" triangle.

3. Assemble the "Paper Dice" according to the directions on the "Paper Dice" page in this section of the guide.

4. Shuffle or mix all the cards together (including the blank cards.)

5. Place the cards face, or writing-side, down near the game board.

6. Each player receives 3 "Skip Pieces."

How To Play:

1. The player whose birthday is first among the group of players will begin the game. (Or, create another way to choose the first player.) Then, players will take turns in a clockwise direction.

2. On his or her turn, each player rolls the "Paper Dice." Then, the player moves his or her "Playing Piece" the number of spaces displayed on the dice. A player may move his or her "Playing Piece" in any direction during the game.

What To Do On:

"Share a Feeling" Spaces: The player picks a "Feelings Card" and responds aloud to the fill-in-the-blank sentence written on the card. (*Do not write answers on these cards.*) The card is then placed at the bottom of the card pile.

If the player selects a blank "Feelings Card," he or she *writes* a secret fill-in-the- blank "Feelings" sentence on the card. The card is then placed at the bottom of the card pile.

"Go To (   )" Spaces: The player moves his or her "Playing Piece" to the designated space on the game board. The player then shares a feeling or thought about that specific topic or theme. *Remember: responses or answers must relate to your sibling's death.*

"Bridges": The player shares a positive way he or she has changed since your sibling's death OR the player describes something positive which happened since your sibling died.

"Blank" Spaces: The player keeps his or her "Playing Piece" on the blank space until his or her next turn.

Special Area

"Counseling": A player may choose not to roll the "Paper Dice" during his or her turn. Instead, a player may move his or her "Playing Piece" to the "Counseling" area. While in the "Counseling" area, a player may ask any other player for advice OR a player may ask any other player a question. *Remember: advice and questions must relate to your sibling's death or to the player's life since your sibling died.*

Rules of "Survival"

1. Players may choose not to respond to certain questions or "Feelings Cards." During his or her turn, a player may choose not to share his or her thoughts and feelings. The player may then place a "Skip Piece" on the "Skip Pieces" space located on the game board. Once a player uses all of his or her "Skip Pieces," he or she may not skip any more turns.

2. Players are encouraged to relate their responses, their thoughts and their feelings to your sibling's death in some way OR to their lives since your sibling's death.

3. After a player has completed his or her turn, other players may respond to the same question or "Feelings Card." *Remember: Do not interrupt a player during his or her turn.*

The "Game of Survival" is similar to your life as a survivor, because:

- the game has no "end" or "finish"; you will always be a survivor!

- during the game, your "Playing Piece" may land on certain areas or spaces repeatedly, so you may respond to or talk about themes, topics, and feelings many times; as a survivor, you may feel the same emotions during different times in your life. You may experience some of the same issues throughout your life, too. Hopefully, you will have new understandings about the issues and about your emotions as you grow older.

FEELINGS CARDS (Do not write on these cards.)

Anger

I feel or felt angry about

_____'s death
name of sibling who died

because _____.

I think it is _____'s fault

that _____ died.
name of sibling who died

When I feel or felt angry about

_____'s death
name of sibling who died

I _____.

A healthy way to express anger is

_____

Shock/Panic/Overwhelm

The feeling of shock is like

_____

I feel or felt most panicked about

_____'s death when
name of sibling who died

_____.

When I feel or felt overwhelmed about

_____'s death, I
name of sibling who died

_____.

The "It's Not Fair" Feeling

> Since _____ died,
>   name of sibling who died
>
> when I see other siblings together, I feel
>
> _____.

> It's not fair that _____,
>
> because _____.

> Sometimes I think _____'s
>   name of sibling who died
>
> death is unfair, and I wish _____.

Denial

> Once, I _____ed, because I did not want
>
> to believe that _____ died.
>   name of sibling who died

> I didn't believe _____ died,
>   name of sibling who died
>
> because _____.

> Feeling denial for a long time is unhealthy,
>
> because _____.

Sadness

Describe three things you miss about

_____.
name of sibling who died

When I feel or felt sad about

_____'s death, I
name of sibling who died

_____.

I feel or felt most sad about _____'s
name of sibling who died

death when _____.

Joy/Happiness

Since _____'s death, I feel or felt
name of sibling who died

joyful or happy when _____.

When I think about _____
name of sibling who died

I feel joyful or happy, because _____.

_____ and I felt joyful or happy
name of sibling who died

together when we _____.

Guilt

> The feeling of guilt is like
> _____.

> When I feel or felt guilt about
> _____'s death, I
> name of sibling who died
> _____.

> I have felt guilt about _____'s
> name of sibling who died
> death, because _____.

Afraid

> One of my fears about _____'s
> name of sibling who died
> death is or was
> _____.

> I can share my fears about _____'s
> name of sibling who died
> death with _____.

> When I feel or felt afraid about
> _____'s death, I
> name of sibling who died
> _____.

98 / LETTERS FROM A FRIEND

BLANK FEELINGS CARDS (You may write on these cards)

PLAYING PIECES

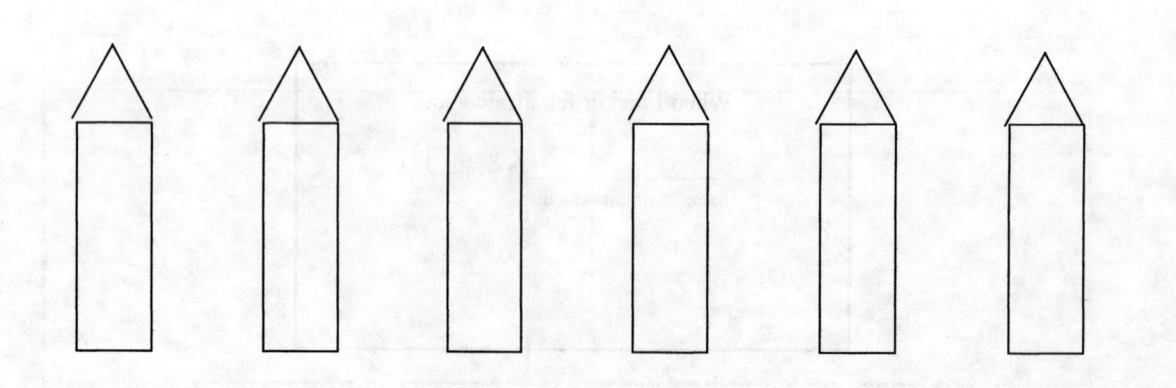

SKIP PIECES

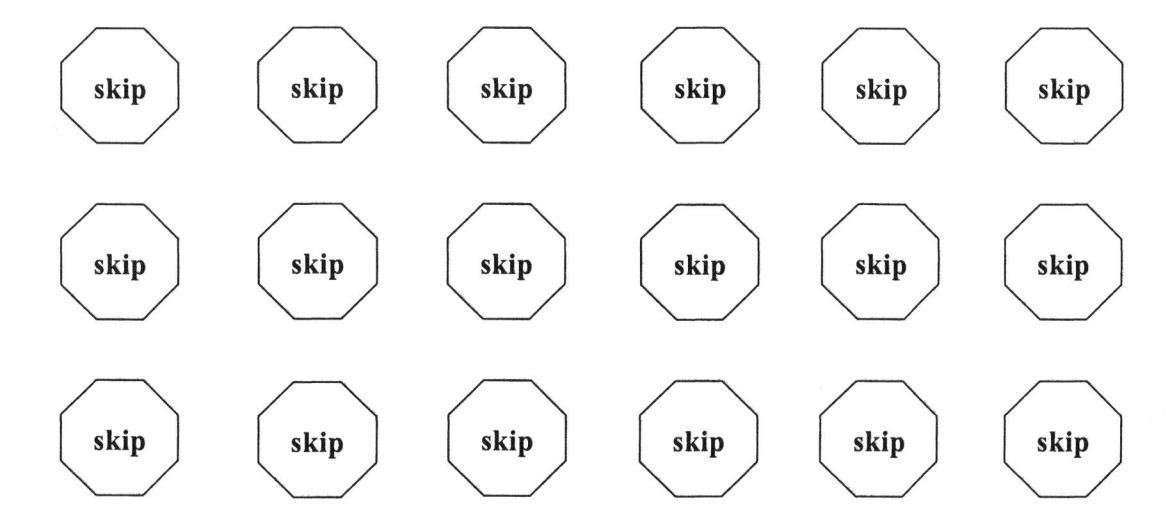

skip	skip	skip	skip	skip	skip
skip	skip	skip	skip	skip	skip
skip	skip	skip	skip	skip	skip

PAPER DICE

Directions:

1. Use scissors to clip around the "Paper Dice."
2. Then, fold along the lines marked "fold."
3. Secure the "Paper Dice" together with tape.
4. On each side of the "Paper Dice," write a "1" or "2."

My Family

MY FAMILY: PARENTS/CAREGIVERS

After my sister died, I was the only child in my family. My mom and dad felt confused about their parenting abilities. In some ways, I believed that my parents were rewarding me for surviving, and being the daughter who lived! I was given Andrea's allowance and the chance to move into her large bedroom. My parents even permitted me to buy a stereo and do other things which Andrea was not permitted to do.

When we were younger, my parents wanted to protect Andrea and me from dangerous or bad things (as most parents want to do for their children). After my sister died, though, my mom and dad seemed to be over-protective. They told me,

> "You're the only child we have now. We want to be very careful nothing bad will happen to you, like it did to Andrea."

My parents expected me to obey their new "rules." They were rules that my sister never had to obey. I was told to call home, at least once, whenever I went out with my friends. My curfew was 11:30 PM; Andrea never had a curfew. During my senior year in high school I wanted to be a foreign exchange student and go to school in Australia. I wanted to learn about another country, like my sister did during her summer college semester in Germany. My parents simply told me,

> "No, you can't go to Australia."

My parents didn't understand that their over-protection **was** *a bad thing happening to me.*

I even had new responsibilities after Andrea died. I did my chores and the chores Andrea used to do. I felt confused about some of my responsibilities, like when my parents told me,

> "You have to be both Erika and Andrea now."

So, I studied more. Instead of going out with friends on weekend nights, I stayed home with my mom to watch her favorite television programs. I played catch with my dad once each week, like Andrea used to do. I did many things my sister used to do.

I tried to be both Erika and Andrea so that my parents would stop missing Andrea, so that my mom and dad would stop thinking about Andrea's death. I believed that I had to be both daughters, and I had to be both daughters *perfectly*.

> "You are the only reason that we are alive," my parents told me.

Me? I was a 15-year-old and I was responsible for my parents' lives? I felt alone and afraid and emotionally weak.

> The responsibilities weren't fair.

How have your relationships with your parents or caregivers changed since your sibling's death?
Write:

<u>Before My Brother/Sister Died</u>　　　　　　　<u>After My Brother/Sister Died</u>

Write a letter to your parents or caregivers about the changes.

> Remember:
> You do not need to give your letter to anyone.
> Just writing may help you feel better.

> Remember:
> It is O.K. for parents and caregivers to cry. Crying is part of healthy grieving. You do not need to be emotionally strong for anyone!
> If you want to . . . cry with your parents or caregivers.

Dear _____,

Responsibilities and Rewards

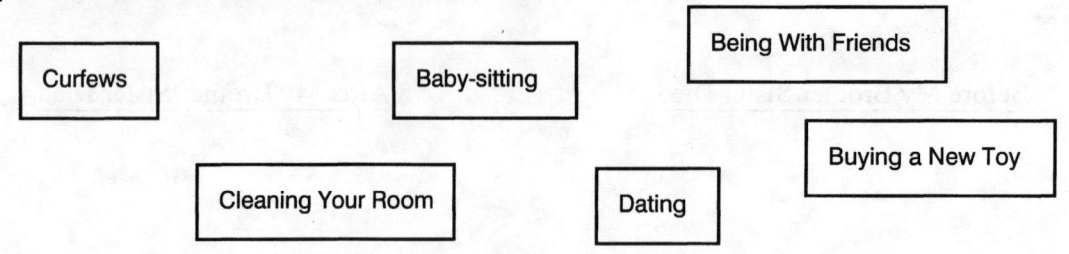

> Curfews
>
> Baby-sitting
>
> Being With Friends
>
> Cleaning Your Room
>
> Dating
>
> Buying a New Toy

After your sibling's death, your relationships with your parents or caregivers may change. You may have new or different responsibilities. Your parents or caregivers may change the privileges you had before your brother or sister died.

Complete this activity with your parents or caregivers.

<u>My Responsibilities</u>

Things I was told or expected to do
Before My Brother/Sister Died

Things I am told or expected to do
Since My Brother/Sister Died

<u>My Privileges</u>

Things I was able or permitted to do
Before My Brother/Sister Died

Things I am able or permitted to do
Since My Brother/Sister Died

> Remember:
> New responsibilities and privileges should be fair to you and to your parents or caregivers!

MY FAMILY: OTHER MEMBERS

After your brother or sister's death, your family members will have their own special ways of grieving. Sometimes, you may feel worried about a family member. You may feel concerned about the way a family member is grieving. Sometimes, you may feel worried about what a family member is doing or saying or how a family member is living.

Do you feel worried about a family member? Write a letter to that person. In your letter, share the reasons for your concern. Also, share ideas or ways to help your family member.

> Remember:
> You may share your letter with your family member, with an adult you trust, or just with yourself.

MY FAMILY CHANGES

A few years after Andrea died, my parents divorced. My dad moved out of our house and into a small apartment in a nearby town. My mother worked more hours at her job so that the house bills would still be paid.

I used to blame Andrea for these changes. I thought my sister's death caused my parents to divorce and also caused my life to be so different. I believe now that many of the changes would have happened even if Andrea was alive.

The changes were even good in some ways. After the divorce:

- my parents stopped arguing;
- both my parents spent more time with me, instead of spending time arguing with each other;
- my mom and dad both smiled and laughed more (I stopped trying to make them feel happy).

Sometimes I feel sad that these changes did not happen sooner. I feel sad because we all waited until the most difficult time in all our lives, Andrea's death, before trying to be a healthy family again.

> Remember:
> Every family is different. The changes that happened in my family since my sibling died, may not happen in your family since your sibling died. Speak with an adult you trust about the changes in your family.

There may be many changes in a family when a family member dies.

Family Trees

On each tree branch . . .

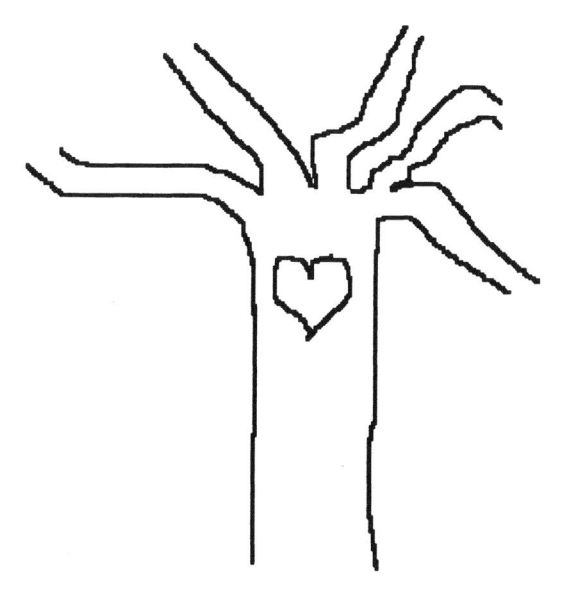

BEFORE
Your Sibling Died

Write something about each person in your family.

AFTER
Your Sibling Died

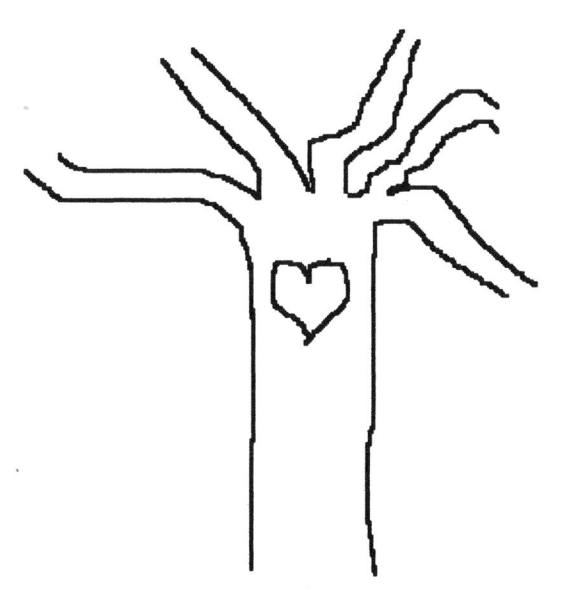

How did each person in your family change?
Write about the changes on each tree branch.

Remember:
Some changes in your family may have happened, even if your brother or sister did not die.
Speak with an adult you trust about the changes.

MY RIGHTS IN MY FAMILY

I have the right to:

1. Be loved, because I'm *me*! I should not be compared to my brother/sister who died or to anyone else!

2. Make mistakes. I know that my brother/sister who died *was not* perfect either.

3. Talk or cry about my brother/sister who died.

4. Celebrate growing older!

5. Live my own life and plan my own goals. I can feel happy. I can laugh. I can have my own wonderful experiences!

What other "rights" do you have in your family?
Write:

6.

7.

8.

9.

10.

Share your "rights" with your family members.

MY SIBLING QUILT

A quilt is a special blanket made from patches of different types of fabric squares. Some quilts are designed with a theme or topic, and each patch square represents something special about that topic.

Design a paper quilt about your brother or sister who died. You may design each special patch square yourself, or give a paper square to your family members or other people who knew your brother or sister, and ask them to design it! When all patch square designs are completed, tape the patch squares together to form your special "sibling quilt." Some patch square design ideas include: memories of your sibling who died, your sibling's accomplishments, hobbies or his or her favorite things. You may use drawings or words within your designs.

> Remember:
> You may also create your quilt from fabric patches. The fabric patches can be sewn together to make your "sibling quilt." Ask an adult to help you with the sewing project.

MY FAMILY: SIBLING SURVIVORS
(My Brothers/Sisters Who Are Alive)

Inside each frame below, draw a picture or place a photo of your surviving siblings. You may design other frames if you need to.

Think about how each of your surviving siblings has grieved since your brother's or sister's death. On the lines below each picture or photo, write three words that describe your surviving sibling's grief.

Write a letter to one or to each of your surviving brothers/sisters.

In your letter, you may describe your feelings about him or her. You may share the things you like about your surviving sibling. You may also describe the kind of sibling relationship you would like to have with your surviving brother or sister since your sibling's death.

> Remember:
> Share this activity with an adult you trust before sharing it with your surviving brother/sister.

Since your brother or sister died, there are many ways you can be involved in sibling-like activities, even if you have no surviving siblings.

- Volunteer at a hospital pediatric unit
- Be a teacher's helper after school or during summer school
- Baby-sit
- Work or volunteer at a recreation center, day care center, or summer camp

What other ways can you be involved in sibling-like activities?
Write about your ideas inside the frames.

MY FAMILY: NEW SIBLINGS

Once family members have experienced healthy grieving of your sibling's death, welcoming new brothers and/or sisters to your family may be positive events.

Since your sibling's death, do you have any new brothers or sisters?

Inside each frame below, place a photo or draw a picture of your new siblings. You may design more frames if you need to.

_____

Sibling's Name

This sibling was welcomed into my family on

_____.

Date

_____

Sibling's Name

This sibling was welcomed into my family on

_____.

Date

_____

Sibling's Name

This sibling was welcomed into my family on

_____.

Date

Even if your new brother or sister is unable to read, write a letter to him or her.

In your letter, you may describe your brother or sister who died. You may also share your feelings and the things you enjoy about your new sibling.

> Share this activity with an adult you trust before sharing it with your new brother or sister.

> You may keep your letter and share it with your new sibling when he or she is able to read.

> If you have more than one new brother or sister, you may use additional sheets of paper to write more letters.

Police and the Law

POLICE INVESTIGATIONS AND COURT TRIALS

Sometimes, if a death happens suddenly or if a person caused a death to happen, there may be a police investigation and/or a court trial. During police investigations and court trials, law officials try to understand why a death happened. They may also try to punish a person who caused a death to happen.

Surviving family members, caregivers and friends may be so involved in police investigations and/or court trials, that they may not experience healthy grieving.

"**Your Right To Grieve**" is a game which may help you if there are or were police investigations and/or court trials about your sibling's death. While playing the game, you may better understand police investigations and/or court trials and also feel more comfortable sharing your grief feelings. You may play the game with people you trust, who are aware of or participate in the police investigations and/or court trials about your sibling's death OR you may play the game with yourself.

During the game, players may substitute the term "sibling" with their own relationship to your brother or sister.

"**Your Right To Grieve**" is on the following page.

Playing Pieces

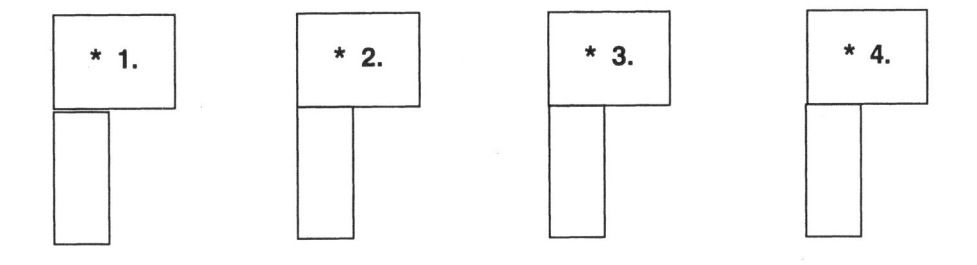

| * 1. | * 2. | * 3. | * 4. |

114 / LETTERS FROM A FRIEND

YOUR RIGHT TO GRIEVE
Read the previous page titled "Police Investigations and Court Trials" before playing this game.

If someone caused your sibling's death, what punishment do you think the person should get? Draw a picture about it.	Tell or write about a person involved in the police investigation or court trial whom you dislike or disliked.	Think about your sibling who died. Say a positive thing about your sibling's life.	Write two words that describe the police investigations and/or court trials.
Draw a picture of your sibling who died. When you are finished, describe each part of your drawing.	****************** ****************** ****************** ****************** ******************		Draw a picture that portrays something special about your sibling who died.
Describe what happened during one day of the police investigation or court trial.	_____ _____ _____		Think about a time when you laughed together with your sibling who died. Tell or write about it.
What have you learned about police investigations and/or court trials? Draw a picture about it.	Think about a time when you cried together with your sibling who died. Tell or write about it.	How do or did you feel during the police investigation or court trial? Draw a picture about it.	Tell or write about a person involved in the police investigation or court trial whom you like or liked.
Draw a picture of someone involved in the police investigation or court trial. Ask other players to guess who the person is.	\multicolumn{3}{l|}{"Your Right To Grieve" may be played by 1 to 4 players. Players may move their "Playing Pieces" in any direction. Players may continue playing the game for as long as they choose. *You will need:* blank pieces of paper crayons or markers scissors dice (you may use the dice in the "Game of Survival" section in this guide) *Preparation:* use scissors to clip the "Playing Pieces" from the previous page. *Directions*: 1. Place all "Playing Pieces" on the gameboard. 2. Players decide which person will begin the game. 3. On his or her turn, each player rolls the dice. The player moves his or her playing piece the number of spaces displayed on the dice. 4. The player responds to the question or completes the activity written on the space. 5. Then, each player shares his or her response or activity with the other players.}		
Describe something you miss about your sibling since he or she died.			
What do you think should have been done differently during the police investigation or court trial? Tell or write about it.			
Place Playing Pieces Here **To Begin Game**			

If you are participating in police investigations or court trials about your sibling's death, you may share your feelings and thoughts about the investigations and trials on this page. You may also describe things you see or hear during the investigations or trials. Add more note pages if you need to.

POLICE INVESTIGATION AND COURT NOTES

What happened today: Date: _____

What happened today: Date: _____

What happened today: Date: _____

Newspapers, Television, and the Media

Sometimes, after a death happens, there may be a death notice or an obituary written in the newspaper. Death notices and obituaries inform many people that a death has happened.

Sometimes, a death notice or an obituary describes the person who died and the details of the person's life. Surviving family members may also have their names printed in a death notice or an obituary.

Besides death notices and obituaries, there may be newspaper articles or television news stories about your brother or sister who died or about your sibling's death.

Write an article or a news story about your brother or sister who died. You may also write a death notice or an obituary about your sibling's death.

> Remember:
> You may share the article, news story, death notice, or obituary with an adult you trust or just with yourself.

> Remember:
> You may also ask an adult you trust to help send the article, news story, death notice, or obituary to the media in your town!

OR

Share your feelings about an article, a news story, a death notice, or an obituary that was completed about your brother or sister who died.

My Sibling's Friends

YOUR SIBLING'S FRIENDS

You may have had special relationships with your sibling's friends before your brother or sister's death. You may have or want to have special relationships with some of your sibling's friends since your brother or sister died.

Continuing or developing your relationships since your sibling's death may help you and your sibling's friends grieve. You may also develop very special friendships or bonds between you and your brother or sister's friends.

Complete this activity with your sibling's friend or friends.

Since your brother or sister's death, plan a monthly outing or activity for you and your sibling's friend or friends to do together. You may plan more outings or activities if each person chooses to.

> Share this activity with an adult in your family.

Together, you may:

- visit the place where your sibling's body is;
- go to a place which was one of your sibling's favorites;
- go to religious services;
- go to movies or sports events;
- go for walks or exercise.

Month   **Date**   **Outing/Activity**

> Remember:
> During your outings or activities, it is O.K. to talk or not to talk about your brother or sister who died.

LETTERS FROM A FRIEND

Since your brother or sister's death, write a letter to one of your sibling's friends.

> Remember:
> You do not need to share your letter with anyone.

> Remember:
> You may use additional sheets of paper to write to other friends.

TO MATCH OR NOT TO MATCH

Since your brother or sister's death, complete this activity with one of your sibling's friends.

You will need:
    blank sheets of paper
    markers, crayons or colored pencils
    scissors

> Remember:
> You may copy the lists for additional people to participate.

Directions:

1. Use scissors to separate the two lists.
2. Keep the list titled, "My Sibling" for yourself. Give the list titled, "My Friend" to your sibling's friend.
3. For each item on the list, each person draws a picture related to that topic or theme.
    Do not share your drawings with anyone until all topics or themes have been completed.
4. After all topics or themes on the list have been completed, participants may share and discuss their drawings with each another!

My Sibling	*	*My Friend*
Draw a picture of:		Draw a picture of:
Topic/Theme	*	Topic/Theme
1. Your sibling's favorite hobby or thing to do	*	1. Your friend's favorite hobby or thing to do
2. Your sibling's favorite color		2. Your friend's favorite color
3. One of your sibling's talents	*	3. One of your friend's talents
4. One of your sibling's "bad" habits		4. One of your friend's "bad" habits
5. The best thing about your sibling	*	5. The best thing about your friend

Use scissors to clip around the drawings. Then, make a collage: paste or tape the drawings on the next page!

> Remember:
> Participants may decide to draw pictures about additional topics or themes.

6.   6.

7.   7.

8.   8.

"THE BROKEN CLOCK"

One of my sister's high school classmates gave birth to a baby boy last month. Two of my sister's friends are married now. Some of her other friends have bought their own homes. Some are moving to live in other states. All of Andrea's friends are still living.

Sometimes I feel sad and I wonder: What would my sister be doing if she was alive?

Where would you be now, Andrea?

Would you have gotten well and earned that degree?
Teaching second grade children,
Or those in grade three?

Would you live on your own,
In some far away land?
Or be married and have children, just as you planned?

Would you be in my wedding, as I would in yours?
Would we be friends or fight each other in "sibling wars"?

Would I be an aunt to a baby niece or nephew?
Would I help decorate baby's room in shades of pink or light blue?

There are people your age whom I often have seen,
And I wonder how life with you just might have been.

Since you have died, I've survived. I've continued living my life somehow . . .
But I still can't help but wonder where you'd be
now.

LETTERS FROM A FRIEND

Since your brother or sister died, what do you think about and how do you feel:

- when you see your sibling's friends as they grow older?
- when you see people who are the same age as your brother or sister would have been if he or she was alive?

Write about your thoughts and feelings in a poem.

> Remember:
> Poems do not always rhyme.

Written by: _____

Dreams and Nightmares

It may be late at night or during an afternoon nap . . .
. . . maybe early one morning . . .

you've been sleeping and dreaming . . .
. . . dreaming about your brother or sister who died.

Sometimes, you may feel frustrated, angry or sad after waking up and remembering your dream about your brother or sister. While you were asleep, you may have dreamt that your sibling was alive again. Yet, when you awaken, your dream may seem to be more of a nightmare, when you realize your brother or sister truly *is* dead.

Sometimes, you may feel afraid to sleep, because you do not want to dream about your sibling who died.

> Remember:
> All of these feelings are O.K. to feel. Many people feel frustrated, angry, sad—even afraid after dreaming about their siblings who have died. Sharing your dreams with an adult you trust may help.

Other times, you may feel happy when remembering dreams about your sibling. Since his or her death, you may feel comforted to dream about your brother or sister.

Describe or draw a picture of a dream you have had about your brother or sister who died. Share your feelings about your dream.

DREAM SAVER

Since my sister died, I've had many dreams about her. I've dreamt that Andrea is, once again, alive and healthy. Many times I've felt sadness and anger after remembering my dreams because when I awoke, I was reminded that my sister truly had died.

So, I invented my "dream saver." I'm not sure how I invented her, or when I first encountered my dream saver. I do know that whenever I am dreaming about Andrea, my dream saver interrupts my dream.

She says, *"Erika, you're asleep. You're dreaming that your sister is alive, but Andrea truly is dead."*

I awake after hearing my dream saver's voice. I feel less sad and angry about the reality of my sister's death, because I was reminded of her death *during* my dream instead of *after* my dream. In a way, my dream saver "saves" me from some emotional pain.

Most times now, I feel happy after dreaming about Andrea. I realize that memories of my sister truly are part of me. I know that each dream, in a very special way, helps me understand and adjust to Andrea's death. Each dream helps me experience again the joys of my sibling relationship.

You may feel or have felt sad, angry, frustrated, or afraid after dreaming about your brother or sister who died.

Create your own "dream saver."

Draw a picture of:
your *Dream Saver.*

How will your dream saver "save" you during a dream about your brother or sister who died?

DAY DREAMS

I've imagined that I stayed home with Andrea instead
of going to work with my mom the day Andrea died.

I've thought about arriving home earlier that day and finding Andrea inside the garage **before**
she got inside the car to die.

I've imagined Dad's car using all its gas, the engine stopping, and the poisonous fumes vanishing **before**
Andrea could breathe the fumes and die.

During my day dreams, I save Andrea's life. I change the events which happened on December 17, 1983—the day *my sister died*. I have the control to make my sister be alive and healthy again . . . for awhile.

Day dreams are dreams, though. I am reminded of the reality:

Andrea is dead.
December 17, 1983 cannot be changed.

Because . . .
I didn't stay home with Andrea and
I didn't arrive home earlier and
The car didn't use all its gas.

And I can't change anything that has already happened.

You may day dream about your brother or sister who died. You may imagine changing the events which happened before your sibling's death.

> Share this activity with an adult you trust.

Draw pictures about your day dream. You may add more scenes if you need to.

Dream Scenes

Scene 1

Describe:

Scene 2

Describe:

Scene 3

Describe:

Scene 4

Describe:

Anniversaries and "Firsts"

Anniversaries are like bookmarks within time: they mark the important and special days in your life while time passes.

Anniversaries are especially important after your sibling's death, because you are reminded that time *is* passing and that you *are* truly surviving your brother or sister's death.

There are many anniversaries during the days, weeks, and months after your brother or sister has died. Some of these special and important days may be called "firsts." It may seem difficult to celebrate "firsts," because they often happen soon after your sibling's death. During "firsts," you may be reminded of your brother or sister's death.

> Since your sibling's death, "firsts" may be difficult for you to do. Doing "firsts" is important and may help you live your life again! Sometimes changing the ways you used to do things when your sibling was alive may help you cope with "firsts" since your sibling's death.

Since your sibling's death, write the dates you "first":   <u>Date</u>

- did something you used to do with your sibling when he or she was alive _____

    What did you do? _____

- slept in your bed _____

- ate food _____

- went to school _____

- laughed _____

- did something you enjoyed doing _____

    What did you do? _____

Write about and record other "firsts":   <u>Date</u>

Think about your favorite holiday or other special day which you celebrated with your sibling while he or she was alive.

Draw a picture about your memory.

Inside the frames below, paste or tape photos of holidays, birthdays, family trips, and other celebrations you shared with your sibling while your brother or sister was alive. Below each photo describe your memory of the special event. You may use additional pages to design more frames if you need to.

ANNIVERSARIES AND HOLIDAYS: CELEBRATING AS A SURVIVOR

> Remember:
> Since your sibling's death, it is O.K. to think about and to share your memories of past family celebrations.
> It is O.K. to think about the times your brother or sister celebrated with your family.
>
> Since your sibling's death, it is also important to create new memories of holidays and other special days . . . and to celebrate them as a
> *survivor!*

Since your brother or sister's death, describe how you would like to celebrate or how you celebrated:

> Share your plans with your family!

	Date/Year:	Celebration:
Christmas:	_____	
Hanukkah:	_____	
New Year's:	_____	
Easter:	_____	
Passover:	_____	
Halloween:	_____	
Independence Day:	_____	
Father's Day:	_____	
Mother's Day:	_____	
Valentine's Day:	_____	
Your Sibling's Birthday:	_____	

Add other holidays and special days to your list:

CELEBRATING YOUR SIBLING

There may be many dates which were special during your sibling's life. Since your brother or sister's death, there may also be dates which are special or important to you.

Planning and participating in rituals or activities are ways to help celebrate all the dates which are special to you. Rituals and activities may also help you celebrate your brother or sister's life.

Rituals and activities may include:

- Donating a gift to the hospital on the anniversary of the date your brother or sister was diagnosed with an illness or injury.
- Planting flowers on your sibling's birthday. Then, donating the flowers to a nursing home or charity.
- Volunteering to help with religious services at your church, temple or other special place on the anniversary of the date your brother or sister died.

Write about dates which are or might become special or important to you since your sibling's death. Then, plan a ritual or an activity to help celebrate that date and to help celebrate your brother or sister's life.

> Remember:
> There are many rituals and activities which not only help celebrate your sibling's life, but benefit other people, too!

> Share this activity with your family!

Special or Important Date   Ritual or Activity Planned

DEATH ANNIVERSARIES

Like other anniversaries, death anniversaries are like bookmarks, too. The death anniversary marks the day your brother or sister died. Throughout your life, the death anniversary may be difficult to celebrate. The way you choose to celebrate the day your sibling died may be different each year. Sometimes, you may try not to think about your sibling's death on the anniversary. Other years, on the death anniversary, you may decide to go to the place where your sibling's body is, attend religious services or participate in activities you enjoy. You may choose to think about your sibling's death and to remember how you felt on that day—

>the day your brother or sister died.

Plan to celebrate your brother or sister's death anniversaries. Think about, then describe, a special ritual or an activity you may want to do on each death anniversary in memory of your sibling's life!

> Share your plans with an adult you trust.

Death anniversary: Celebration:

1st year

2nd year

3rd year

4th year

5th year

6th year

7th year

8th year

9th year

10th year

On one of your sibling's death anniversaries, write a letter to your brother or sister who died. In your letter, describe your thoughts, feelings, and accomplishments since your sibling's death. You may then read your letter aloud to your brother or sister who died.

> Remember:
> You do not need to share your letter with anyone!

Identity

WHO AM I NOW?

So, who am I since my sister died?

Who am I since:

      I can't imitate Andrea anymore?
      I can't learn from my sister's advice and
                            examples anymore?

Who will:

      be my friend when I feel lonely?
      be my protector when I am teased at school?
      be my sister, when I need one? *(And I always need one.)*

I don't know how to do so many things.
How will I:

      decide where to go to college?
      choose classes, choose boyfriends,   choose?

Who will tell me:

      "Don't quit."
      "Things will be O.K."

or even . . .   "Stop being a bratty sister."

Who will I become when I grow "older," when all I've known is how to be "younger"?

                Who?

DIFFERENT SIMILARITIES

My sister and I were alike in many ways. I discovered similarities between us, even after Andrea died. Andrea enjoyed, and I enjoy:

- laughing
- creative writing
- traveling
- pets
- helping people

While my sister was alive, we noticed that our lips formed the same shaped frown whenever we were concentrating on a project. Our eyes had the same almond shape. Our hands and fingers looked identical.

Yet, there were many differences between my sister and me. The differences did not make either of us "better" than one another. The differences simply made us . . . different.

Andrea	I
enjoyed being away from home	enjoy being at home
did not share her feelings with people	share my feelings with people
wore sheer stockings, leather boots, and high heels	wear cotton socks, denim skirts, and hiking boots
wanted to work in a school	worked in a hospital
did not survive the last time she tried to die	am surviving Andrea's death

136 / LETTERS FROM A FRIEND

Think about the similarities and differences between you and your brother or sister who died. Then, complete:

> **Remember:**
> The similarities and differences help make you a unique person! You are loved for who *you* are!

My sibling and I were alike, because:

My sibling and I were different, because:

Interview three people who know you and who knew your sibling before he or she died. Ask each person to describe the similarities and differences between you and your brother or sister.

Similarities	Differences

THE SIBLING QUESTION

Do you have any brothers or sisters?

Since my sister's death, I used to answer "No" to that question. I used to tell people that I was the "only" child in my family.

I felt guilt after telling people that I had no siblings. I knew that I had lied to them, because I truly believe that Andrea will always be my sister, although she is no longer a physical part of my life.

In some ways, I chose not to acknowledge my sibling relationship, because I didn't want to be different from other people whose siblings were alive. By not acknowledging Andrea's death, though, I was also not acknowledging her life.

I now realize that I <u>am</u> different from people whose siblings are alive.

I have a special appreciation of sibling relationships.
I have had to question myself about the kind of person I am and the kind of person I want to be; I can no longer imitate my sibling's example.
I have learned about myself as I have worked through my grief.
I have a special goal to help other sibling survivors.
I have gained emotional strength.

I appreciate life because I have survived a death.

And . . . I would never surrender one of my differences just to belong to a group of people or to be more like someone else.

This is me.

> You may share this activity with an adult you trust.

What if:

1.
You are at a party.
You meet someone whom you think is cute.
He or she asks, "Do you have any brothers or sisters?"

You answer, "*Yes,*"   You answer, "*No*," because
and tell the person about your sibling who died, because

2.
At school, your teacher tells the students to write about their families.
Do you write about your brother or sister who died?

Yes, because   *No*, because

3.
A classmate's brother dies in a car accident. No students or school staff talk with your classmate about his or her sibling's death. Do you share your experience about your sibling's death with your classmate?

Yes, because   *No*, because

Since your sibling's death, how are you different from your friends or from people who are your age? Describe the strengths, feelings, beliefs, and understandings you have since your brother or sister's death. You may write a letter to one of your friends or to people your age about your differences.

> Remember:
> You do not need to share your letter with anyone.

Celebrate You.

Emotional Support

RELAXATION

Read, then practice doing this relaxation exercise! You may even read aloud and record this exercise with a tape recorder. Then, press the "play" button and listen to the exercise!

Find a place where you will not be disturbed while you practice this relaxation exercise. You should also feel safe and comfortable while you are in the place. You may lie down or sit during this exercise.

Gently, close your eyes.

Imagine your body is floating a few feet above the place you are now.

Feel your head, your shoulders, your stomach and legs moving, gently, side to side.

Your body is hovering in the air. You feel safe, as your body gently sways, side to side, in the air.

Now, imagine your body is floating higher into the air. You know you are safe as your body rises.

You feel your body gently moving side to side in the air.

Your body is floating to a special place. You feel safe and calm as you float to your special place.

Relax as your body gently sways, side to side, to your special place.

Relax and imagine being in your special place.

You control your body as it floats in your special place.

Stay in your special place for awhile.

Notice the things you see and hear, taste and touch in your special place.

(Pause for a few minutes.)

You are going to leave your special place now, but you know you can come back later.

Your body gently moves, side to side, floating safely in the air.

Your body slowly moves back, through space and time...back to the place you are now.

Gently, your body sets down. You feel relaxed and comfortable.

Slowly, count to 10, and open your eyes.

You are loved.

COUNSELING/EMOTIONAL SUPPORT

Since my sister's death I've gone to five different counselors. Each counselor taught me something about myself. Yet, until counselor #5, I didn't feel as if I was working through my grief about Andrea's death.

I chose to go to counseling, because I felt sadness and guilt about my sister's death for a very long time. I didn't know how to express my grief feelings or how to cope with the changes in my life since Andrea died.

I tried to share my feelings and thoughts with my family, but they seemed busy working through their grief, too. My friends tried to help me. They listened to me and sometimes cried with me, but I knew they couldn't truly understand or help me with my long term grief. Afterall, none of my friends were professional counselors.

Five different counselors. Maybe, during the years I went to counseling, my emotional needs changed so I changed counselors. Sometimes I think that I went to so many counselors, because I never felt satisfied or happy with their services. Afterall, even though the counselors could listen, advise me and emotionally support me, none of them could do the one thing I truly wanted—to make my sister alive and healthy again. Each counseling experience was special though. Each experience, I know, helped develop the person I am today.

During one of my last counseling sessions, I was told to go home and write a "good-bye letter" to my sister. It was the most difficult homework assignment I had ever completed.

I sat in my home, on the sofa, staring at a blank piece of paper. Although I believed, as I believe now, that my sister's spirit and her memory will always be with me, I knew Andrea's physical body died.

I began to write. Two hours later, I had completed five pages. I felt emotionally tired, yet also peaceful. Within that letter, I had shared with my sister love, sadness and a very special "Good-bye."

On the following page are some thoughts from that letter.

September, 1992

Dear Andrea,
I know I will never physically see you again—not the way I used to. Your brown eyes. Your frizzy hair. The bump on your nose . . .

. . . I want to say so many things to you: Why did you choose to die and leave me?
. . . I miss you so much . . . There's a part of me—inside me—it still feels empty. . . .

I miss your puppet shows . . . and watching you getting ready for your dates . . . and hearing you play your violin. . . .

We could have created so many more memories together. Someday . . . I could have held your baby. I could have been at your wedding . . . you're supposed to be at mine . . .
Sometimes, I feel so deserted.

There are times when I look in the mirror or at photographs of myself, and I see the same features you had. And I feel special. . . .

I need you to help me when I feel confused, to protect me when I feel afraid, to love me when . . . always.

Who will help me, protect me, and love me since you died? *Me. I'll always have myself.*

Thank you for the games of tag . . . for letting me swim in the pool during "adults-only swim" . . . for telling me that the red balloon had the penny prize inside it at Donna's birthday party.

Please know, when you were inside the garage dying, that I loved you. (Even though I only told you "I love you" on Christmas Day.) I never understood, until you died, that you were my best friend, too. I'm sorry I never told you so many important things. . . .

. . . My life will be different since you died. The house is quiet. Parts of me are quiet, too . . .
We are still sisters. I believe your spirit is a part of me-always.

I was blessed and lucky to have you as my older sister those 15-1/2 years . . . and still now . . . forever. . . .
I love you. . . .
On the night before your death, you said to me, "Good-night."
Good-night, my sister.   Good-bye, Andrea.

Always, your younger sister, Erika

Sometimes, and especially if your sibling died suddenly or unexpectedly, you may not have said, "Good-bye" to your brother or sister. You may not have shared many of your thoughts and feelings with your sibling before his or her death.

Write a "Good-bye" letter to your brother or sister who died.

> Remember:
> You may read your letter at or near the special place where your sibling's body is. You may also share your letter with someone you trust or just with yourself.

EMOTIONAL SUPPORT CHOICES

At times, you may not understand your feelings. During times like these, it is especially important to share your feelings and thoughts with someone you trust. It may be helpful to speak with friends or your family.

Sometimes, friends and family may not understand your feelings especially if they have never experienced sibling death. Many times, friends and family are not able to understand your feelings, because they are trying to understand their own feelings about your sibling's death.

There are many other people to share your feelings with and different ways to share your feelings.

- Support Groups: are groups of people who are having or have had experiences like yours! At support groups, people meet together to share their thoughts and feelings. There are many support groups for siblings whose brothers and sisters have died. Ask a counselor, school social worker, or hospital social worker about these special groups.
- Counselors and Social Workers: are people who may also help you share your grief emotions. There may be counselors and social workers at your school, at hospitals, and in the community where you live. Usually, the thoughts and feelings you share are "confidential" so the counselor or social worker cannot tell anyone else.
- Religious People: include priests, nuns, reverends, rabbis, and chaplains. If you have questions, especially about your religion or your god, religious people may help you. Many religious people are also good listeners and may help you understand your thoughts and feelings better.

Reading books about your sibling's cause of death or about surviving your sibling's death may also offer you emotional support.

> Remember:
> If your grief feelings are not shared or expressed in healthy ways, your grief will not simply go away. Sometimes, unexpressed grief feelings may cause other problems to happen even years after your sibling's death.

Whatever type of emotional support you choose, find a person whom you can trust or a program in which you feel emotionally safe.

> Remember:
> Good emotional support services will not suddenly help you solve all your problems or instantly help you stop feeling your grief emotions. No emotional support service can make your sibling be alive and healthy again. You must do your own grief work and find the special solutions to many of your own problems. Emotional support services should emotionally support you, as you help yourself!

As you work through your grief, you may try many different kinds of emotional support services. You may try, as I tried, many different styles of the same type of emotional support.

> Remember:
> There is no time limit to emotionally heal after your sibling's death.

You do control your grief. Although you may feel afraid, choose to trust and love people again after your sibling's death. Decide to develop emotionally close relationships since your brother or sister died.

Choose to truly be a survivor!

EMOTIONAL SUPPORT DIARY

On this page, begin a special "emotional support" diary. Add additional diary pages if you need to. After each meeting with your emotional support person or after each support group session, write about it! Describe your feelings about the meeting or session.

After several meetings or sessions, read your emotional support diary again.
Notice the ways *you are surviving*.

> Remember:
> Throughout your life, it is O.K. and healthy to ask for and get emotional support!

BREAK TIMES

There may be times when you want to stop thinking about your sibling's death. You may want to stop feeling your grief emotions, for awhile.

Think about the ways you would like to "get a break" from thinking about your brother or sister's death or from feeling your grief emotions. Use scissors to clip pictures from magazines which describe or portray the ways you would like to "get a break."

Paste or tape the pictures on this page.

> Remember:
> At times, it is O.K. to stop thinking about your sibling's death. It is healthy to "get a break" from feeling your grief emotions, for awhile. Your grief work will not "go away" during the break times. You will still need to work through your grief when the break is finished.

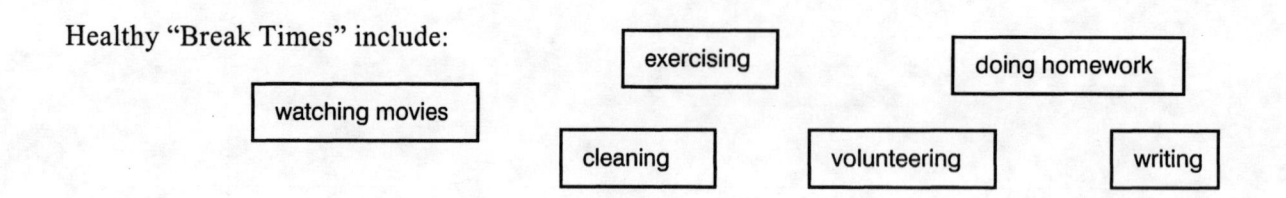

Healthy "Break Times" include:

- watching movies
- exercising
- doing homework
- cleaning
- volunteering
- writing

"ESCAPING" GRIEF

You can not escape your grief after your brother or sister's death.
After a death happens, some people try to escape their grief by drinking alcohol, running away from home, taking illegal drugs or doing other unhealthy things.
Your grief is part of you. You can not truly escape from it, because you can not escape yourself.
Learning to understand and work through your grief is more healthy and will help you live—instead of avoid or delay—your life again!
Speak with an adult you trust if you think you are trying to escape your grief or if you are doing dangerous things.
You deserve to survive today!

GET-A-BREAK COUPONS

Use these coupons when you need extra emotional support!
Use scissors to clip out each coupon. Blank coupons are for you to design.
Give the coupons to your family and other people you trust.

Coupon for: *I need a hug.*
Date used: Given to:

Coupon for: *I would like to go out with friends.*
Date used: Given to:

Coupon for: *Please make this for dinner tonight:* _____
Date used: Given to:

Coupon for: *I want to talk with you.*
Date used: Given to:

Coupon for: *I don't want to talk with you now.* We can talk with each other on/at _____
Date used: Given to:

Coupon for:
Date used: Given to:

Coupon for:
Date used: Given to:

Coupon for:
Date used: Given to:

148 / LETTERS FROM A FRIEND

DOOR SIGN

Write your own messages in the blank spaces on this door sign.
Use scissors to clip out the door sign and arrow.
Use a paper fastener to attach the circle on the arrow to the circle on the door sign.
Position the arrow toward whichever message you choose.
Post the door sign on the door to your own private space.

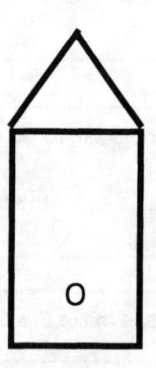

I'M SLEEPING

_____   _____

I'M USING THE PHONE   COME IN

                              O

I WANT TO BE ALONE   _____

I'M DOING HOMEWORK   _____

I'LL BE OUT OF HERE IN _____ MINUTE(S)

Surviving My Future

MY SPECIAL CELEBRATION

Weddings　　　　　ELECTIONS　　　Parties　　　　School Plays

Getting your license　　　Dances　　**Birthdays**

Graduations　　　　　　　　　Religious Events

Since your sibling died, think about a day which was or will be special or important to you. Write a letter to your brother or sister who died. In your letter, describe the special or important day. Share your thoughts and feelings about the special or important day.

> Remember:
> You do not need to share your letter with anyone.

> Remember:
> It is O.K. and healthy to celebrate the special and important days of your life!

REMINDERS

There may be times when you are reminded of your sibling who died. You may see, hear—even smell—things and think about your brother or sister who died. Sights, sounds and smells like these may be called "reminders."

I think about my sister when:

• I see people wearing college state sweatshirts, because Andrea was a college student when she died.
• I hear violin music, because Andrea played the violin.
• I smell the scent of the perfume Andrea gave as her last Christmas present to me.

You may use pictures, photographs, or words to complete this activity.

I am reminded of my brother or sister who died when . . .

I see this:

I hear this:

I smell this:

Describe other times you are reminded of your brother or sister who died:

RAINBOWS

Some people believe that there are "good" things about the "bad" things which happen in life. It may seem difficult to think of anything "good" about your sibling's death. After a death happens, some "good" things may be:

- developing even more emotionally close relationships with family and friends;
- learning about your strengths as a survivor;
- helping other survivors cope with a death and with their grief.

Inside each "color" of this paper rainbow, describe something "good" about your brother's or sister's death.

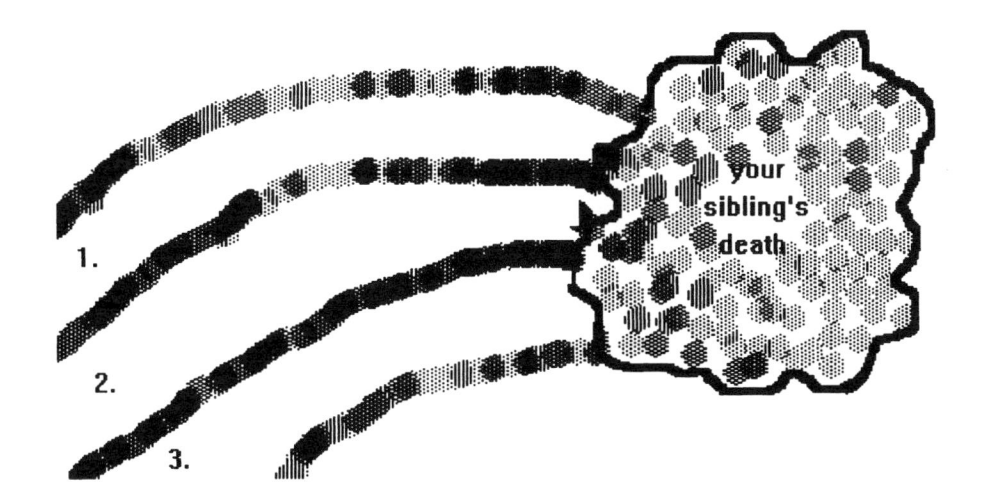

1.
2.
3.

your sibling's death

You are shining past that dark cloud!

Write a "thank you" note to your brother or sister who died. In your note, describe the things you have learned about yourself and about life because of your sibling's death.

> Share your note with an adult you trust!

Thank You!

Shapes of Survival: A Game of Reflection

> You may play this game with family members or by yourself.

Directions:

1. Use scissors to clip out the paper shapes.
    The paper shapes are on the page titled, "Paper Shapes," page 155.

2. Place all paper shapes in a pile.

3. During each player's turn, he or she selects a shape from the top of the pile. The player then locates the matching shape on the game board.
    The game board is on pages 156 and 157.

4. The player then responds aloud to the direction or question near the matching shape.

5. After a player responds to the direction or question, he or she receives an "O" for that corresponding shape. "O's" may be tallied on the "O" sheet.
    The "O" sheet is on the page titled, "O Sheet," on page 154.

6. The shape is then placed at the bottom of the pile.

O SHEET

> You may make copies of this sheet and play "Shapes of Survival" again!

Each player receives an "O" after responding to a direction or question near a shape. Players receive one "O" per shape. If a player selects a shape repeatedly, he or she may respond to the corresponding direction or question again (and does not receive an additional "O") or wait until his or her next turn.

Players may choose not to respond to a direction or question. Then, however, the player does not receive an "O" for that shape.

"Shapes of Survival" is completed once every player has had a chance to select each shape and respond to each corresponding direction or question on the game board.

Everyone is a survivor!

Shape	Player Number	1	2	3	4	5
key						
star						
heart						
tree						
circle						
cross						
cloud						
lips						
rectangle						
triangle						
rainbow						

PAPER SHAPES

Use scissors to clip out these paper shapes.

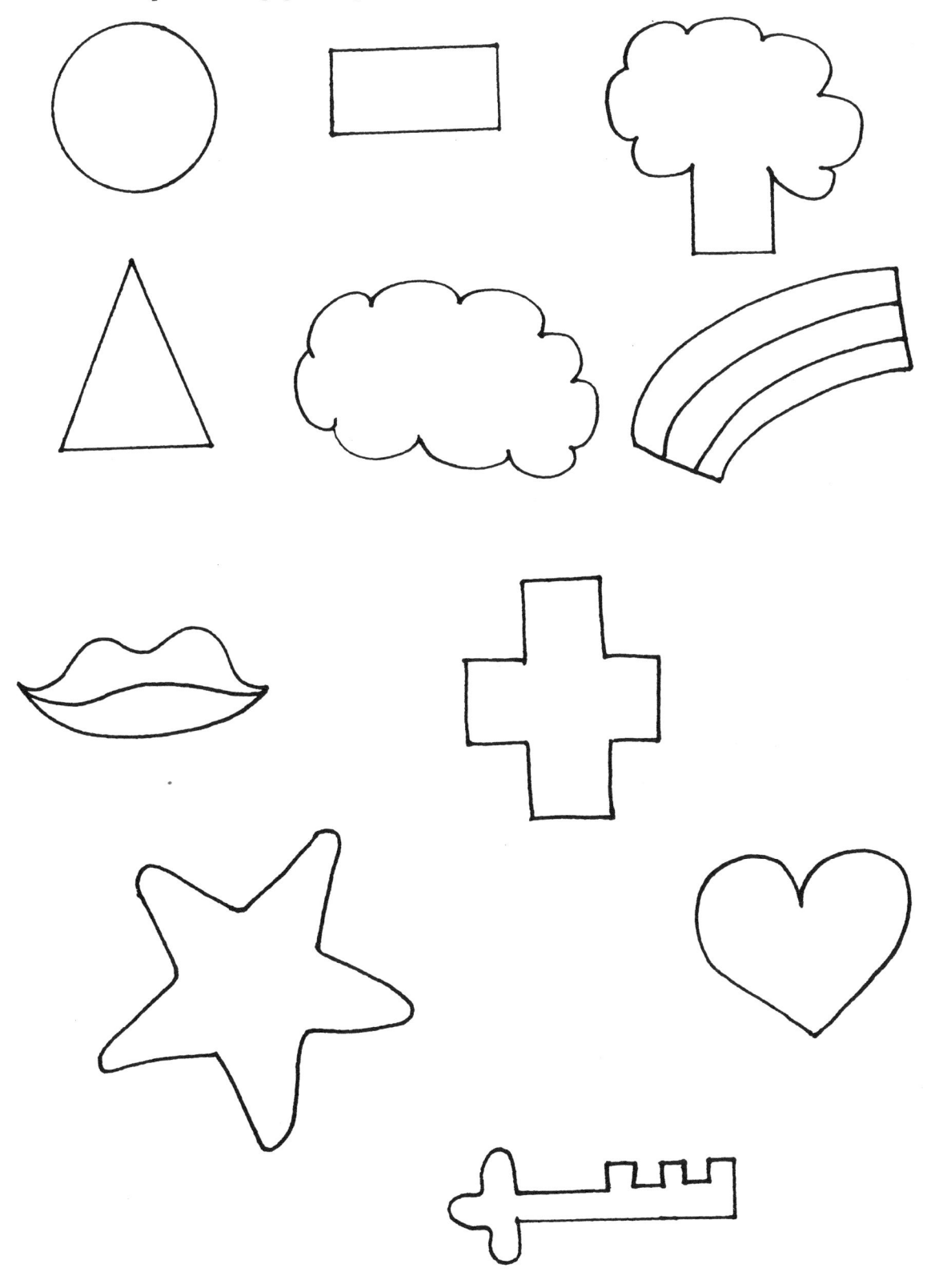

156 / LETTERS FROM A FRIEND

GAME BOARD

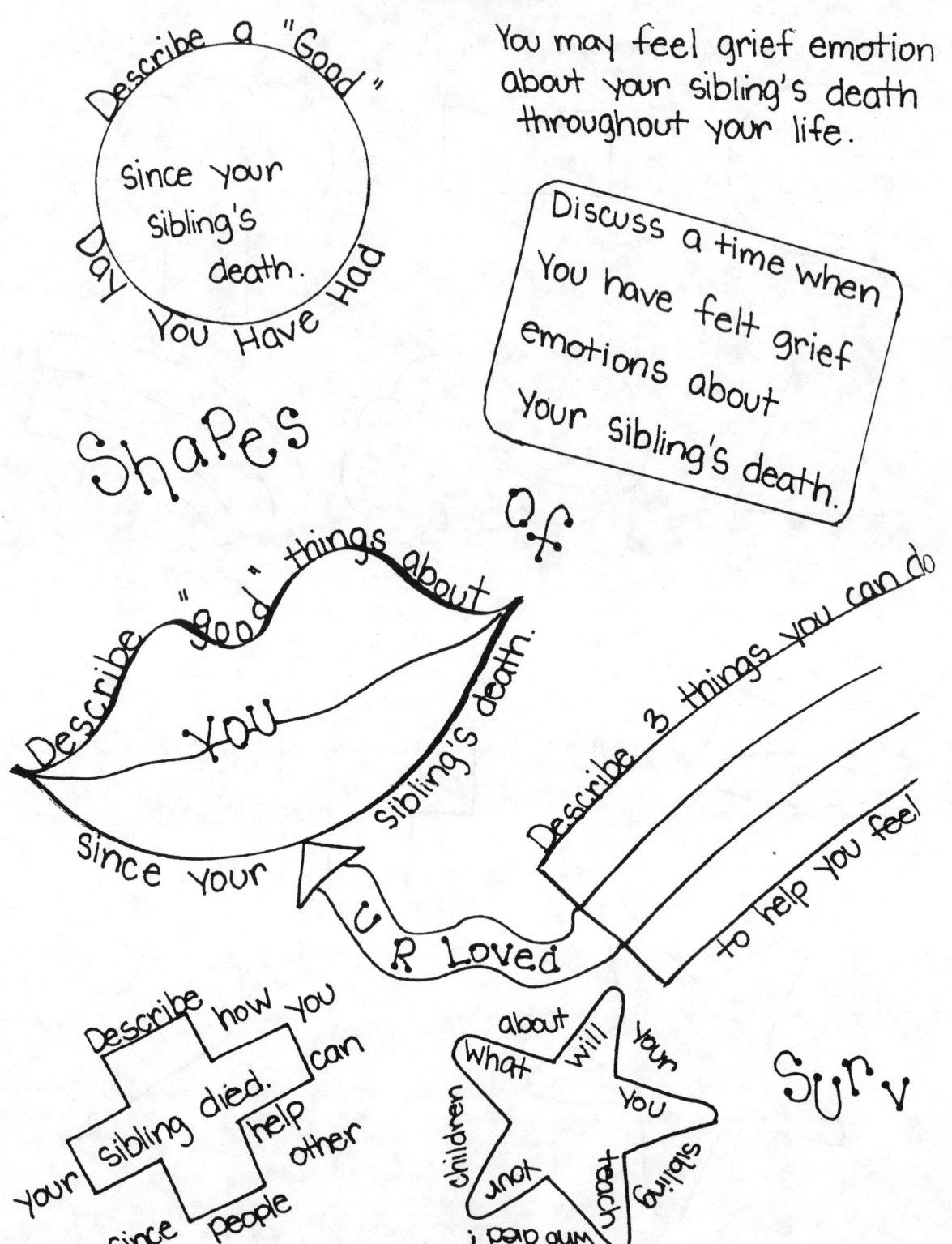

Describe a "Good" Day You Have Had Since your Sibling's death.

You may feel grief emotion about your sibling's death throughout your life.

Discuss a time when you have felt grief emotions about your sibling's death.

Shapes

Describe "Bad" things about you since your sibling's death.

Of

Describe 3 things you can do to help you feel U R Loved

Describe how you sibling died. can help other Since people

what about will your you teach your sibling who died? children

Surv

GAME BOARD

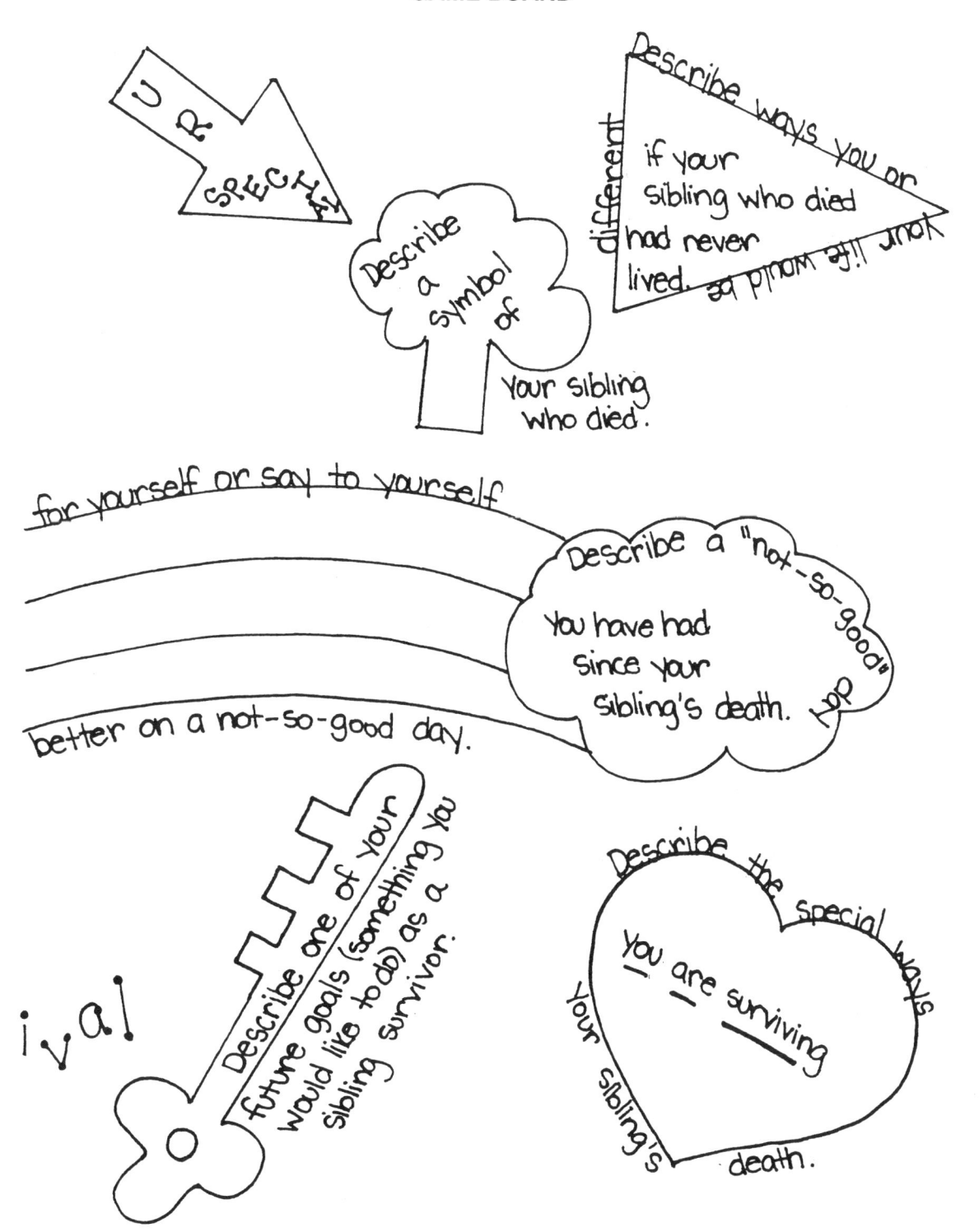

- U R SPECIAL
- Describe a symbol of your sibling who died.
- Describe ways you or your life would be different if your sibling who died had never lived.
- (rainbow) for yourself or say to yourself ... better on a not-so-good day.
- Describe a "not-so-good" day you have had since your sibling's death.
- ¡viva! Describe one of your future goals (something you would like to do) as a sibling survivor.
- Describe the special ways you are surviving your sibling's death.

Forgiveness

When my sister died, I felt angry with many people. I felt angry with my god. Mostly, I felt angry with myself: I felt guilt.

Andrea has not been a physical part of my life for many years now. During these years, I have learned that I can not grow emotionally if I do not work through my anger and my guilt. I have also discovered that before I can even try to forgive those with whom I have felt angry, I must first forgive myself.

And so, as an adult, I now forgive myself as the 15-year-old with whom I've felt so angry since Andrea's death.

I felt angry with myself, because I	I forgive myself, because I
always tried to be more beautiful, smarter, or more loved than Andrea, even after she died.	realize we both compared ourselves to each other. We weren't better than one another—just different from each other, and just as beautiful, just as smart, just as loved!
said and did nasty things to Andrea while she was alive.	realize most siblings say and do nasty things to each other. We also said and did nice things to each other. Nasty and nice things are parts of healthy sibling relationships.
didn't tell Andrea "I love you" more often while she was alive.	realize our family didn't verbally express our love for one another. I expressed my love for Andrea whenever I did or said nice things to my sister. I have learned to verbally express my love for people since Andrea's death. I have improved my relationships with people.
didn't stop Andrea's death from happening.	cannot control other people or their lives. Andrea chose to die. I choose to live.
lived.	deserve to feel happy. I deserve to accomplish my goals, to live my life, and to survive Andrea's death.

I forgive you, Erika.

Find the activity titled, "Mirror Talking." The activity is in the "Guilt/If I Had Only" on page 74. Complete the "Mirror Talking" activity before continuing.

Review the reasons you have felt angry with yourself about or since your sibling's death.

Then . . .

For each reason, write a response and forgive yourself.

> Share this activity with an adult you trust.

I have felt angry with myself, because   I forgive myself, because

Forgive Yourself. You are loved!

Since your brother or sister's death, there may be many reasons you have felt angry with yourself.

Write a letter to YOU. In your letter, describe the special ways you forgive yourself.

> Remember:
> You may share your letter with someone you trust or just with yourself.

Since your sibling's death, you may have felt angry with someone or something. You may blame or have blamed someone or something for your sibling's death. At first, it may seem difficult to forgive the person or thing, but forgiving may help you emotionally heal and grow as a survivor. Forgiveness does not mean you will ever forget your sibling or how and why he or she died. When you stop feeling angry about your sibling's death, you may start to feel happy about your life.

When you are ready and choose to emotionally heal and grow as a survivor, write a letter to someone or something with whom or with what you have felt angry. In your letter, describe the special ways you forgive the person or thing.

> Remember:
> You may share your letter with the person or thing or just with yourself.

Pen Pal Program

WELCOME TO THE PEN PAL PROGRAM

This program is just for children and teens who are coping with their siblings' death.

Throughout this guide, you have been invited to write letters and notes within many activities. Some of your letters and notes may have been written to family members, friends, strangers—even yourself! You may have decided to share the letters you've written or you may have chosen to share them just with yourself. All of the letter writing activities are designed to help you share your thoughts and feelings in healthy ways.

The pen pal program is another way to help you share your thoughts and feelings. Also, it is a way to develop friendships with other children or teens who have also experienced sibling death. Each time you write a letter or note to your pen pal, you will be emotionally supporting someone special. And, when mail is delivered to your home, remember to look for your pen pal mail!

To join the pen pal program, complete and mail the application form and the consent form. The forms are on the following pages.

PEN PAL PROGRAM APPLICATION FORM

This form must be mailed with the Pen Pal Program Consent Form. Your application will not be processed without the completed consent form.

Date: _____

Your Name: _____

Your Age: _____

Your Sex: (male or female) _____

Your Address: _____

City: _____ State: _____ Country: _____ Zip Code: _____

Your Phone Number (for Pen Pal Program files only): (_____) _____
                                                                             area code

Describe your brother or sister who died:

My brother/sister died, because:

When did your sibling die? month: _____ day: _____ year: _____

I would like a pen pal who is similar to me in: (please mark your choice(s) with an X)

                                                _____ age

                                                _____ sex

                                                _____ sibling death experience

                                                _____ other (describe another similarity)

Please note that attempts to accommodate preferences will be made, but are not guaranteed.

164 / LETTERS FROM A FRIEND

PEN PAL PROGRAM CONSENT FORM

This form must be mailed with the Pen Pal Program Application Form. Your consent form will not be processed without the completed application form.

You must be at least 18 years old to complete your own consent form. Pen pals who are 17 years or younger must have a parent or legal guardian complete the consent form.

Use scissors to clip the dotted line.

— —

I, _____, am the pen pal and am at least 18 years old, or I am the
    please print your name

parent or legal guardian of _____. I hereby give consent to <u>Erika</u>
    please print name of pen pal applicant

<u>Barber</u> to process the enclosed Pen Pal Program application form and to include the applicant in this program. I understand the purpose of the Pen Pal Program is for surviving children and teens to emotionally support one another following sibling death. I understand the personal information (with the exception of phone numbers) on the application form will be shared with designated pen pal participants for the purpose of establishing pen pal relationships. Therefore, on behalf of the pen pal applicant, I hereby and irrevocably waive all rights to privacy and publicity as it relates to the Pen Pal Program.

<u>Erika Barber</u> acts solely as a forwarding agent and does not verify any of the information provided by participants in this program, nor can <u>Erika Barber</u> guarantee any results from participating in this program. In addition, <u>Erika Barber</u> has no control over the actions of individuals participating in this program. In consideration for the applicant's participation in this program, I hereby release <u>Erika Barber</u> from all responsibility for any arrangements I or the applicant might make through the applicant's participation in this program, and expressly waive any claim or cause of action against <u>Erika Barber</u> for any reason pertaining to the applicant's participation in this program.

<u>Erika Barber</u> reserves the right to edit any application for participation in this program and reserves the right to refuse any application.

    I HAVE READ, I UNDERSTAND, AND I AGREE TO ALL OF THE ABOVE.

Signed: _____
    please sign your name

Your relationship to the Pen Pal Program Applicant: _____
(If you are completing this form and you are also the Pen Pal Program Applicant, you must submit proof that you are 18 years or older. For example, a photocopy of your driver's license or other identification which states your age.)

Date: _____

Completed and signed consent and application forms may be mailed to <u>Pen Pal Program</u>.

    The address is on the dedication page of this guide.
    Thanks for your friendship!

Parents, Caregivers, and Professionals

TIPS ON UTILIZING THIS GUIDE WITH THE CHILD OR TEEN AUTHOR

As a parent, caregiver, or professional, it is important to convey to the child or teen author that he or she and his or her thoughts and feelings are important and special. Children and adolescents engaged in this guide should be reminded that all emotions are okay and healthy to feel when a sibling is sick, injured, dying, or after sibling death. You may also reinforce the concept of healthy and acceptable expressions of emotions as you introduce many of the activities within this guide.

Before beginning any activity or discussion with the child or teen author, practice these suggestions:

- Be aware of and share your own feelings and thoughts related to the sibling's illness, injury or dying/death situation. If you are unable to express your thoughts and feelings in beneficial ways with the child or teen, find a supportive adult with whom the child or teen feels comfortable. Remember, it is okay and healthy to cry with the child or teen.

- Remember that each child or teen expresses his or her emotions in special ways. Grief emotions, especially, may be expressed at different times throughout the child or teen's life as his or her understanding and thought processes mature and as the child or teen's special developmental milestones occur.

- Allow adequate time to introduce guide concepts and to engage authors in the related activities or discussions. Also, select an environment with limited noise and interruptions prior to beginning an activity or discussion.

- Reassure the child or teen author that you or a designated supportive adult will be available to answer questions, participate in discussions or listen as he or she speaks about the sibling's illness, injury, or death.

While engaged in the guide activities or discussions with the child or teen author, remember to:

- Be truthful, honest and sensitive when explaining concepts related to sibling illness, injury or death.

- Use language and terminology which encourage the child or teen to comprehend the concepts. Avoid ambiguous or unclear words and phrases.

- Remember that healthy expression of thoughts and feelings may be verbal or nonverbal. Do not force the child or teen author to share completed activities or his or her emotions.

- Be aware of the child or adolescent who is not practicing healthy expression of emotions and thoughts. Remember, you are not emotionally weak to ask for professional help for yourself or for the child or teen.

WAYS I CAN HELP THE CHILD OR TEEN AUTHOR

> Complete this activity with the child or teen author.

1.

2.

3.

4.

5.

6.

7.

8.

9.

10.

Daily Schedule

Within this guide, there are activities that require a blank schedule. Make copies of this blank schedule.

Day of the Week: _____

GOAL OR THING TO DO

Time

6:00 A.M. _____
    6:30 A.M. _____
7:00 A.M. _____
    7:30 A.M. _____
8:00 A.M. _____
    8:30 A.M. _____
9:00 A.M. _____
    9:30 A.M. _____
10:00 A.M. _____
    10:30 A.M. _____
11:00 A.M. _____
    11:30 A.M. _____
12:00 Noon _____
    12:30 P.M. _____
1:00 A.M. _____
    1:30 P.M. _____
2:00 P.M. _____
    2:30 P.M. _____
3:00 P.M. _____
    3:30 P.M. _____
4:00 P.M. _____
    4:30 P.M. _____
5:00 P.M. _____
    5:30 P.M. _____
6:00 P.M. _____
    6:30 P.M. _____

Evening Activity:

168 / LETTERS FROM A FRIEND

Within this guide, there are activities that require a blank calendar. Make copies of this blank calendar.

SUNDAY	MONDAY	TUESDAY	WEDNESDAY	THURSDAY	FRIDAY	SATURDAY

Quilt, sibling, 107

Relaxation exercises, 140
Religion/God, 47-51, 144
Reminders of deceased sibling
 activities to do to help deal with sibling's death, 150
 belongings of sibling, 64-65
 faces and voices of strangers, 56, 150

Sadness
 empty space inside body, 66
 friends, deceased sibling's, 121
 Game of Survival, 96
 healthy grieving, part of, 53
 miss about sibling, writing about things you, 68
 music, 69-70
 reasons for, writing about, 96
Safe place, feeling afraid and visiting a, 80-83
School after death of sibling, returning to, 42-46
Scream therapy, 58
Shapes of Survival Game, 153-157
Shock, 94
SIB-A-THY sympathy cards, 36-37
Sign-in books at death services/ceremonies, 32
Similarities/differences between deceased/surviving sibling, 135-136
Social workers, 144
Songs, 69-70
Soul of deceased sibling, 51
Suicide, 20
Support groups, 63, 144
 See also Emotional support
Survivor, being a
 break times (stop feeling for a while), 146-148
 death wished for in order to stop grief emotions, 70
 differences between surviving sibling and peers, 139

[Survivor, being a]
 future, surviving the, 149-152
 Game of Survival, 92-99
 good-bye letter to deceased sibling, 141-143
 Shapes of Survival Game, 153-157
 See also Family, the
Sympathy cards, 35-38

Television, 116
Thank you note to deceased sibling, 152
"Think of Laura" (Cross), 69

Unfair/it's not fair, 71-73, 95

Wake, the, 28-29
Words/phrases used to explain death, 18
Writing
 acknowledgment/celebration of dead sibling's life, 131
 day your sibling died, 22
 death services/ceremonies, 34
 God/religion, 48
 good/positive things, 76
 joy/happiness, 89
 memories of deceased sibling, 84
 past death experiences, 17
 pen pal program, 162-164
 real/believable, when/where does death become more, 56
 sadness, 67
 thank you note to deceased sibling, 152
 unfair/it's not fair, 73
 See also Letter writing; Poetry

Your Right To Grieve Game, 113-114

Index

Acknowledgment/celebration of dead sibling's life
  anniversaries and holidays, 130
  Game of Survival, 96
  joy/happiness, feeling, 88-90
  planning, 131
  school after death of sibling, returning to, 46
  telling others about sibling's death, 137-138
Activities to help deal with sibling's death
  calendar, activity, 9
  differences/similarities between deceased/
    surviving sibling, 136
  door sign for break times, 148
  dying sibling, with, 8-9
  friends, deceased sibling's, 119
  Game of Survival, 92-99
  good about your sibling's death, describing
    something, 151
  memories of sibling, 85
  mirror talking, 75
  painting feet/hands of sibling, 25
  paper person, designing a, 3
  planning, 131
  quilt, sibling, 107
  reminders, 150
  scream therapy, 58
  sibling survivors, 108-110
  sympathy cards, 38
  telling others about sibling's death, 138
  Your Right To Grieve, 113-114
  See also Drawing pictures; Letter writing; Poetry;
    Writing
Afraid, feeling
  forgetting, fear of, 83-86
  Game of Survival, 97
  less afraid, feeling, 87
  place sibling died, visiting, 86
  safe place, visiting a, 80-83
  talking about death, 18
Alcohol/drugs, groups against driving under
  influence of, 63
Andrea's story/death (author's sibling), xii,
  19-20

Anger
  belongings of deceased sibling, 64-65
  courtroom, imaginary, 59
  displacement, 58
  drawing pictures, 61-62
  forgiveness, 158-161
  Game of Survival, 94
  guilt, 74
  letter writing, 60
  poetry, 57
  scream therapy, 58
  support groups, 63
Anniversaries and firsts, 128-133
Appearance of sibling when death occurs, 10, 24

Belongings of deceased sibling, 64-65
Body of deceased sibling, 23-25, 39-41
Books read for emotional support, 144
Break times (stop feeling for a while), 146-148

Calendar, activity, 9
Cancer awareness groups, 63
Caregivers, surviving sibling's relationship with,
  100-102, 104
Caregivers helping child/teen authors to utilize
  this guide, x, 165-168
Celebrations of important days since sibling died,
  149
  See also Acknowledgment/celebration of dead
    sibling's life
Cemetery, visiting the, 39-41
Counseling/counselors, 92, 141, 144
Court trials, 59, 113-115
Cremation, 40
Crying, 53, 69

Daydreaming, 126-127
Day your sibling died, writing about, 22
Death anniversaries, 132-133

Death services/ceremonies
  involvement, level of, 31
  memories of, sharing, 33
  past death experiences, 17
  planning, 12-13, 30-31
  sign-in books, 32
  story-poem about, 34
  wake, 28-29
Decorating location of deceased sibling's body, 41
Denial, 54-55, 95
Diary writing, 27, 145
Differences between surviving sibling and peers, 139
Differences/similarities between deceased/surviving sibling, 135-136
Displacement, 58
Door sign for break times, 148
Drawing pictures
  anger, 61-62
  appearance of sibling when death occurs, 10, 24
  courtroom, imaginary, 59
  daydreaming, 127
  before death, imagining what happened to sibling, 21
  death services/ceremonies, 30, 33
  dreams and nightmares, 123, 125
  God/religion, 48, 51
  guilt, 79
  hospice care, 7
  hospital setting, 1-2
  letter to dying sibling, 11
  people surrounding sibling when death occurs, 10
  place sibling died, 10, 21
  place where sibling's body is buried/located, 40
  sibling survivors, 108
Dreams and nightmares, 123-127
Driving under influence of alcohol/drugs, groups against, 63

Educational programs, bodies donated to, 40
Emotional support
  choices, making, 144
  counseling, 92, 141
  diary writing, 145
  groups which relate to way in which sibling died, 63
  relaxation exercises, 140
  school after death of sibling, returning to, 43, 45
Envy, 71-72
Escaping grief, 146

Fair, it's not, 71-73, 95
Family, the
  changes within, 104-105
  feelings about sibling's illness/injury, different, 5
  new siblings, 111-112
  other members, 103
  parents/caregivers, 100-102
  quilt, sibling, 107
  rights in the, surviving sibling's, 108
  sibling survivors, 107
Feelings about sibling's illness/injury/death
  diary writing, 27
  family having different, 5
  Game of Survival, 92
  God/religion, 50
  media, the mass, 116
  seeing or hearing sibling who is dead, 56
  visiting place where sibling's body is buried/located, 40
  See also specific emotion/feeling
Firsts and anniversaries, 128-133
Forgetting, fear of, 83-86
Forgiveness, 158-161
Friends, deceased sibling's, 117-122
Future, surviving the, 149-152

Game of Survival
  dice, paper, 99
  directions, 92
  feeling cards, 94-98
  how to play, 92
  preparation, 92
  rules, 93
  skip pieces, 99
  special area, 93
  what to do on:, 92-93
"Garden of Envy, The," 71-72
God/religion, 47-51, 144
Good-bye letter to deceased sibling, 141-143
Grief feelings, 52-53, 146
  See also specific feeling/emotion
Groups which relate to way in which sibling died, 63
Growth (personal) through dealing with sibling's death, 137, 151
Guilt feelings
  anger, 74
  drawing pictures, 79
  forgiveness, 158
  Game of Survival, 97
  good things you have done with/for deceased sibling, write down, 7

[Guilt feelings]
   mirror talking activity, 75
   nice and nasty memories, 77-78
   sharing reasons for, 74

Happiness/joy, 88-90, 96
Headstones, 41
Holidays, 130
Hospice care, 6-7
Hospital setting, 1-2

Identity questions/issues, 134-139
If I had only feeling. *See* Guilt feelings

Joy/happiness, 88-90, 96

Law, police and the, 59, 113-115
Letter writing
   anger, 60
   celebrations of important days since sibling died, 149
   death anniversaries, 133
   to deceased sibling, 11, 68, 141-143
   family members, to, 103
   friends, deceased sibling's, 118
   God/religion, 49
   good-bye letter to deceased sibling, 141-143
   illness/injury, to sibling's, 4
   new siblings, 112
   organizations which relate to way in which sibling died, 63
   school after death of sibling, returning to, 44

Mausoleum, 40
Media, the mass, 116
Medical programs, bodies donated to, 40
Memories
   belongings of deceased sibling, 64-65
   death services/ceremonies, 33
   firsts and anniversaries, 128-133
   forgetting, fear of, 83-86
   joy/happiness, 90
   nice and nasty memories about deceased sibling, 77-78
   similarities/differences between deceased/surviving sibling, 135-136
Mirror talking activity, 75, 159

Music, 69-70

Newspapers, 116
Nice and nasty memories about ᴅ 77-78

Organ donation, 40
Organizations which relate to wa sibling died, 63
Overwhelmed, feeling, 94

Panic, 94
Parents, surviving sibling's relati 100-102, 104
Parents helping child/teen author guide, x, 165-168
Past death experiences, 14-18
Pen pal program, 162-164
People surrounding sibling when
Pets that have died, 14
Photographs
   of dead sibling, 24, 64
   firsts and anniversaries, 129
   hospital setting, 1-2
   letter to dying sibling, 11
   new siblings, 111
   pets that have died, 14
   sibling survivors, 108
Place sibling died, 10, 21, 86
Place where sibling's body is buri 40, 41
PLANET ILLNESS/INJURY, 5
Planning
   acknowledgment/celebration of life, 131
   activity calendar, 9
   death anniversaries, 132-133
   death services/ceremonies, 12-1
   first few days after sibling's dea
   friends, deceased sibling's, 117
   school after death of sibling, retu 43
Poetry
   anger, 57
   death services/ceremonies, 34
   friends, deceased sibling's, 122
   sadness, 70
Police and the law, 59, 113-115
Professionals helping child/teen au this guide, x, 165-168